SIX MILES
PER
HOUR

SIX MILES PER HOUR

PER

HOUR

Patrick McGlade

To order additional copies of this book, contact:
Xlibris Corporation
1-888-795-4274
www.Xlibris.com
Orders@Xlibris.com
96050

CONTENTS

For all the kids who battle arthritis every day

CHAPTER 1

It was the morning of April 23, 2010. I woke up already in my running shorts. I'd been wearing the same pair of shorts for a week because I was used to saving laundry for when I "really needed it."

I reached for my hat and threw it on my head so I didn't have to worry about combing my hair. I had done this for more than three months. It was second nature to wake up and toss my hat on.

As I put my shirt on in the dark, I didn't even stop to see if it was inside out or not. I just sort of hoped and went with it. But in reality, it didn't matter. Once I started running, I'd take it off anyway.

I woke up early that day; earlier than normal. It could've been because this was my normal sleep schedule as of late. Minimal. Not by choice; I just hadn't been able to sleep lately. It could have been a result of my consuming 6,000 calories per day to maintain body mass, and my metabolism was working non-stop. But perhaps it because this was the last day of my run across America and the nerves had my brain more active and my body more antsy than usual.

As I woke up in the hotel room in Savannah, Georgia, a flood of memories rushed my brain and I knew I was up for good. I thought about the morning I started, 112 days earlier, back in Huntington Beach, California. To look ahead and think about what I might see, where I'd go, who I'd meet, what body part might break first—it was, in short, terrifying. Yet, here I was, on the other side of the United States about to run the final leg of this marathon per day journey to raise money and awareness for juvenile arthritis.

I had said that so many times. "Hi, I'm Patrick McGlade and I'm running across the country to raise money and awareness for juvenile arthritis." I started the run as a quest to raise awareness. I wanted to teach people about the hardships that young kids who had arthritis were facing every day. Though, people had taught me what it was to be truly kind and generous. Complete strangers had raised my awareness of how much people are willing to help other strangers.

I was excited to see my family, my friends, and my girlfriend, Katie; but I was also scared. My life, for the past 4 months, had been nomadic: carrying myself across a country on my own feet. I was nervous about going back to real life; looking for a job, looking for a place to live, figuring out what is next for me. The truth is I wanted to keep running. I wanted to turn north or west or south—any direction to keep running. Now I knew how Forrest Gump felt when he got to the ocean and he just turned around.

I went into the bathroom, finished my business and washed my hands. As I washed my hands, I paused in front of the mirror. It'd been a long time since I had really thought about the whole endeavor. I stood there looking at myself. I looked half homeless with my thick curly beard and longer hair. Both were longer than they'd ever been. I was tan, bronze, brown, whatever you want to call it; but I was dark. I had strange tan lines on my forehead from where my hat lived. But I also had an additional patch of tan up by my hairline where my eternally backwards hat looped in the back to give room for the adjustment of head size. The right side of my body was tanner than the left because I always ran east and as long as it was warmer than 45 degrees, I didn't have a shirt on. I noticed the dark circles that had formed under my eyes and they told the story of my sleepless nights. I still couldn't decide if it was a result of the volume of running or if it was the excitement of the finish.

As I looked, I thought about what brought me here. I thought about not only how surprisingly well my feet held up; I still had all my toenails, thanks to my SmartWool socks, but also why I chose running. There are far more efficient ways to cross a country. A plane, for instance? If I had only taken a plane, I would've seen Katie more than once in the past 4 months; and I would've seen my family and friends more than the few times I had.

I also thought about why I started running in the first place. If I had told myself the day I went for that first run in my worn out New Balance lawn mowing shoes that in three years I would run across the United States I wouldn't have believed me. The one question that still rang in my head with no sign of an answer was: why? What made my quest to lose the couple pounds I had gained in my first two years of college an addiction to run distances people don't normally even like to drive? What made me okay with the little aches and pains that go with running longer distances, and learning to figure out which ones to ignore and which ones to deal with? Why was I okay with being by myself for very long periods of time? Why did I like being on this trip as much as I did? And most importantly, why after running thousands of miles were my legs still so skinny?

I had a lot of time to think on the trip. And I asked myself all of these questions and more. But I thought back to my first run and tried to make sense of my running madness. Where had I gone wrong? Who influenced me to do this? Was I put up to this?

As I stared almost uncomfortably at myself I thought back to the beginning.

CHAPTER 2

In August of 2007 I went for a run one day. I think it was just a nice day, and I thought that's what people do on nice days and I could stand to lose a pound or two. I ran about once a week, maybe one mile at a time, maybe two. I don't remember because I didn't keep track. I didn't measure it out, I didn't time it, and I didn't care.

I think I ran a total of 4 or 5 times and then I got a job as a valet at the Medical College of Virginia Hospital. I ran to the cars to pick them up. And I ran from the cars when I parked them. Word around the garage was, the faster you ran, the more likely you were to get a tip. Being a poor college student, I was up for anything to increase the cash flow.

Little by little, I was getting less and less sore after everyday of work. Then I started going for a run every now and then after or before work. I wasn't serious and I still had no idea how far I was running at a time, but it wasn't ever longer than 20 minutes or so.

Then in May of 2008 I went home for a weekend. My mom was sitting at the table reading a newspaper. She pointed out that there was a half marathon the next day; The Marine Corps Half in Fredericksburg, VA. I was going up to Katie's house that night for dinner and told her I couldn't stay too long because I had a race the next day. Needless to say, she was a bit surprised.

The race was the farthest I had ever run and I loved it. I decided that since I could run half of a marathon I should train for the whole 26.2 marathon.

For most people, the marathon, before running one, is a mythical distance with power and a certain air about it that carries with it proof of endurance and strength. The distance had the same meaning for me. In the words of my mom, "I can understand why someone would want to run ONE marathon just to prove to themselves that they can do it and they are strong enough. But why on earth would you keep going?"

I was 19 and training for a marathon. None of my friends had run one, and I was going it alone. I found a book on how to train for one and it was all based on time spent running, not mileage. The book was easy enough to figure out but difficult to stay on because of school, work, social life and a new problem, injuries. Every time I felt a slight pain, I'd stop because I didn't know what to do. The schedule fell by the wayside and I just ran as much as I could and tried to keep as close to the plan as possible. There was, however, supposed to be one really long run of 3 hours. I didn't have a loop that would take that long and I didn't want to run a small loop multiple times for fear that I would come up with some reason to stop the long run early. I decided the best bet was to run 1.5 hours out and 1.5 hours back on a straight road.

The way out went just fine. I was feeling strong and running well. But humans need water. This little fact must have slipped my mind because I didn't bring any. And if I wasn't smart enough to run with water, I surely didn't have any calories with me. Dumb mistake. I crashed on the way back. I got extremely tired and had cottonmouth. My legs weighed around a ton each, and my head was swirling. With one mile to go I was forced to walk. I wasn't even sure I could do that much without falling over. The last mile was one that I had run repeatedly almost every day in my early days of running. Clay Street in Richmond had terrible sidewalks. Cracks that looked more like fault lines in California formed after years of neglect. Where there wasn't cement, old bricks took the place and there was no shortage of missing, broken, or raised bricks from where trees had shoved their roots. I trudged along happy it was dark. I passed in front of people's houses just beyond their waist-high metal fences that marked their personal territory. I hoped no one was on their porch because I didn't want anyone to see me like this. It was embarrassing. When I finally got home I crawled up the stairs and curled up in my bed and immediately started shaking. It was a scary feeling. My roommates, Mitch and Adam, didn't know what happened but they got me water and stayed there until I was sure I was okay. Now, I always carry water with me.

About 2 weeks before the Marine Corps marathon I read about a race. This was no normal "race." This was more like a survival endeavor, a happening that people simply tried their hardest to push themselves past what other people ever wanted to do and keep going. It was called an ultra marathon.

An ultra marathon, by definition, is any distance over a marathon but usually the races are in denominations of 50 kilometers, 50 miles, 100 kilometers or 100 miles. There are also 8, 12, and 24 hour races where the whole idea of the race is who can log the most miles in the predetermined amount of time.

I was in awe. I couldn't believe I was afraid of running a distance that was half or a quarter of what these people could. They were the immortal in my mind. The strongest and most fit people alive; and not just in the physical sense of the word either. They had figured out the secret to turning off the part of their brain that told them to stop running. This miniscule percentage of the population had the mental capacity to convince their minds that they weren't killing themselves slowly and to keep moving forward would be a good idea. I wanted to do it. I needed to be part of that population of "crazy" runners. There was just one thing I had to do before I signed up for a race; run a marathon.

When race day finally came around I felt like I was undertaking something that was far above my level of fitness and far beyond what I was capable of. I wasn't sure I had trained enough, or ate the right thing the night before, or gotten enough sleep. But I knew that it was possible. 35,000 people lined up with me that day. True, not all of them would finish, but I knew it was physically possible. So in my mind, I knew I would finish.

To this day, the end of that race is the hardest thing I have ever done. I hit the wall with a vengeance at mile 20 and struggled through the end. Every mile past 21 seemed longer than the previous. I was sure the miles were uneven. As the finish line approached in the distance I lost all control and went into a dead sprint. Looking back, that was not the wisest decision I've ever made. As soon as I stopped, my vision started to get brighter and brighter. Then it got so bright all the colors ran together and soon turned white. Within 30 seconds of crossing the line I was blind. I just stood there as I heard other people stumble around me. I felt for the metal barrier and grasped it firmly. A Marine came up to me and asked if I needed assistance.

"Assistance? With what?"

"Do you need an escort to the medical tent?"

"Medical tent? What for? My eyes are the only thing not working right now."

With that, I felt my way down the barrier towards the exit. And within 5 minutes, my vision was back. Clear as ever. At that point I looked at my watch to see my time. 3 hours and 41 minutes. To clarify, this is not a fast time for someone my age, and I knew this. College track stars could easily run in the 2 hours and 40 minute range. And the elite marathoners run between 2 hours and 2 hours 20 minutes. Clearly, my time was not what I was happy about. I was, however, happy that I had set a goal and finished it.

In the book, and everything I had read about training for a marathon, it said I was supposed to take one day off for every race mile. A month? A whole month of no running? I had heard lots of stories of people training for a marathon, getting in the best shape of their lives, running the race, and getting out of shape again. Why did it have to end like that? I decided that wouldn't be me. Sure I was sore after running the race but I was starting to learn the difference between soreness and injury; and I was definitely not injured. After 2 days off, I decided to run again. The following weekend I wanted to go for a longer run. I set out that afternoon with no goal in mind. I simply ran east on Route 5 until I got tired, then I turned around and ran home. I got back to my house some 5 hours after I left and had no idea how many miles I had covered. When I drove it the next day I realized I ran over 30 miles.

I was hooked.

Longer running was more relaxing for me. It was more about the scenery and less about the time. As I got more and more engulfed in it I realized I was supposed to be eating while running. So I did. I would take peanut butter and jelly or honey sandwiches, granola bars, cookies, fig bars, Gu (a gelatinous substance specific for endurance sports) anything I had lying around and I would take off for an afternoon run. I figured I was ready to give a 50k a try. I signed up for my first one: the Swinging Bridge 50k. It was put on by the Richmond Road Runners but was on trails out in Bear Creek State Park. It was freezing at the start.—2 degrees Fahrenheit to be exact. It was so cold my Camelback's hose froze solid. No water for me. My feet were completely numb for the first 25 miles; which I guess is a good thing because then I didn't have to deal with any pain. The whole race, I felt like I had a problem with my nose. I would blow my nose and nothing would come out; but I knew the ol' snot locker was full. I would squeeze it and shake my nostrils and try again and nothing. It was the most annoying feeling in the world until I realized what it was. My nose and all its contents were frozen. And every time I blew, it refroze within 3 seconds. Cold.

The only liquid that didn't freeze was Mountain Dew. So that's what I drank. The whole race was run on Mt. Dew and Chips Ahoy cookies. I guess it worked because I won.

I enjoyed it so much I wanted to run a 50 mile trail race. Being a college student and short on funds I was especially happy when I found out I could run the Bel Monte Endurance Run for free. A friend of mine, Dave Snipes whom I had met soon after Swinging Bridge, was in charge of finding a course sweeper. All I had to do was pick up the trail markings and come in last place. I had no problem with this. So I did it.

Saying Dave is an ultra runner is an understatement. He lives and breathes ultra running and anyone in Virginia who runs ultras knows Dave, or at one time or another has been helped by him in a race whether it's giving them a Tums for an upset stomach or sticking with someone who is having a tough time. During most months of the year Dave, or "Sniper" as some call him as a twist on his last name, Snipes, runs an ultra every weekend. It could be a training run that just happens to be at least 50 kilometers; or more often than not, an organized race up to 100 miles. He knows race courses up and down the east coast like the back of his hand, and he never ever forgets a course. Sniper is the person to go to when you want to run a race you haven't done before and want to know the inside story on the race course, where to pick up certain sized water bottles, when to carry a small backpack, or what the temperature will most likely be at that time of year on the mountain. Although he may not be the fastest runner that ever lived, you can bet that he will finish any race he starts—no matter what.

One race was a big turning point for me. The 24 Hour Adventure Trail Race was going to be the first time I was going to run 100 miles. I had run 50 miles 3 times before, but never over. I was nervous because I had no idea what to expect of this distance. I didn't know if I'd fall apart or stay strong. The plan was to run as long as I could and then walk as long as I could and see if between the two, I could manage 24 hours. The course was an 8 mile long trail loop with a road crossing that marked the middle of the loop. There was a small aid station there with water and chips.

24 hours of being awake, running, and on trails gives you a lot of time alone to think. I had an absolute blast out there. One of the loops, I ran with Dave and it was good to run with someone who had had some experience. Our loop was run during the middle of the day when I was starting to question myself. When it got dark, they allowed a pacer or safety runner to run with you. I had

three people lined up. First up would be my dad. He would do one loop with me and then my brother Kevin would pick up a loop. At the end of his loop, my roommate Adam would run as far as he could.

While I was running with Kevin we approached the halfway point of the loop where we would cross the road and I thought I heard accordion music. This being my first time running more than 50 miles, and the fact that I had been running for 14 or 15 hours at the time, I wasn't completely sure how my body would react. I had heard of people hallucinating strange things while running at night during ultras but I was a little nervous, so I didn't say anything to Kevin. Another minute went by and the accordion music continued only louder. Then Kevin stopped and told me to stop. He asked me, "Do you hear that?" I was so relieved to learn that I wasn't hallucinating. We moved quicker toward the very familiar song being played on the squeeze box. Then as we broke through the end of the trail, there on the side of the road was my dad playing the accordion. It was just the pick-me-up I needed. My dad, Desi, has been playing the Irish button accordion since he was in elementary school and the songs he played to us when we were kids are forever imprinted on my brain and eardrums.

At the end of Kevin's loop, I started running with Adam. He told me he'd do one loop definitely, probably two loops, and hopefully three loops. He ended up running three and a half loops, 28 miles on trails in the dark with me. That was his first marathon, and I was there for it. To be honest, I was more excited about the fact that Adam was willing to push himself so hard to be there for me. He had never run for more than 13 miles at the time.

I ended up running 108 miles that day, tying the course record, and at some point during the night I had an idea; sort of an epiphany. The thought entered my head one second and was decided upon the next. It was more of a voice whispering in my ear, but sounded a lot like my own voice. It went a little something like this, "If I can run for 24 hours straight, I'll bet I can run across the United States."

And that was that. I didn't know when in my life I would do it. I didn't know how, or what my starting and finishing points would be. I knew and was one hundred percent positive I would not only start it, but would finish it as well.

CHAPTER 3

With the goal set in my head, I started looking into people who had done it, records, and how it is done. I felt that I did my homework and now all I had to do was decide when I would do it, to talk to my family and friends about it, and most importantly, finish my college years at Virginia Commonwealth University in Richmond, Virginia.

I figured the first person to talk to would be my girlfriend, Katie. I took her out to a Mexican restaurant called, Mexico Restaurant. They really are getting creative with the names of restaurants around the Richmond area. We were eating the normal things we eat at that restaurant and I decided to drop the bomb. I told her I was thinking about running across the country. She simply asked when. Unfortunately, I hadn't decided on that yet. We talked about it all night and she was incredibly supportive. She never once gave me any reason to think she doubted whether I could do it or not. We tossed around ideas about the best time to do it but came up with no solutions.

Next on my list were my mom and dad.

They each have little pieces of life that they need to know for certain before any proposal. My dad is all for adventure, but needs to know that I am going to finish school first. So I was sure to throw that little piece in there before I ran it by him.

My mom actually needs to know a couple of things when it comes to any running endeavor. First, am I going to lose any more weight? Since I had started training for the marathon about a year ago at this point, I had lost 30 pounds. I wasn't overly skinny, and didn't look like I was sickly, just trim and healthy. She thought I was skinny enough, and was always trying to feed me ice cream, cookies, chocolate and other fattening foods. This, in reality, was great. I had no problem coming home every now and then to a smorgasbord of baked goods.

Second, will I be safe? Nope, I refuse to be safe. I am 21 and invincible. That is why I'm planning to run all 2500 miles at once with a blindfold on and no shoes and fire, lots of fire on sticks, just to make things interesting. Of course I'll be safe, Mom.

The third, unfortunately, I had not come up with a proper answer even for myself yet. She wanted to know the very simple question of why. Quite honestly, I did not have an answer for her when she asked this question. I knew it was coming, it always did. She had a strange way of putting things in perspective, and yet, I always seemed to ignore it when it came to physical challenges. At least, that's the way it had been recently. My mom did not try to tell me it couldn't be done, or that I should not do it. She just didn't know what would possess a person to look at a portion of the globe, or at a giant map of the country we live in and think, "I think I'll run across that." I wish I had a reason for her. I wish I had a reason for myself, for that matter. It was my lack of an answer and certainty for the last question that gave my mom the feeling that this thought was just a phase that would run its course and evacuate my system as soon as I heard about some race I hadn't done yet.

This would not be the case.

The more I thought about it, I was fast approaching on the prime time of my life to give this trip a try. I was graduating in December, and did not have a wife or kids, or a job. I wouldn't have to worry about going back to school, or taking too long off from work, and I didn't have to provide for anyone. Having all of these little facts in my head gave me the impression that I should start sooner rather than later. I wanted to start right after I graduated because I am not one to do too well sitting around doing nothing without a job. It would drive me crazy. Since I would graduate in December, I wanted to leave in January. This really narrowed my choices down as far as routes go.

After doing some research I discovered a route that people had run across the bottom of the country; the only region thawed out enough to run across through the winter months. Even better than that, it was the shortest route! Things were looking good already. I decided that since I had family in San Diego I would start there. After looking at what other people had done, Tybee Island, Georgia seemed like a popular ending point, so I decided to end there. I

"Google mapped" it, and it showed me a route. I pressed the "walking" button, and it showed me the running route. I had an Uncle in Dallas, Texas so I moved the little purple line up a little bit from the initial output so I could swoop through and visit with some family there. I had heard 29 Palms, California was a really cool place to see so I moved the line over to go through there. Other than that, I just left the line where it was and started writing down town names and tracing the route on the road atlas I already owned. I tried not to get too excited because I still hadn't told Katie and my parents that I was planning on doing this within the year, and wasn't completely sure what their reactions would be. Also on the list of things to run by them was the fact that I would more than likely be doing this alone. None of my friends had graduated yet, and the ones that weren't in school couldn't take a couple months off of work to drive across the country in a support vehicle. My research had turned up a few people that had done it solo while pushing a baby jogger full of supplies, 3 of which were a group of guys who had run it just the previous year and were generally close to my age. So, the baby jogger was decided upon.

When I started thinking about the fact that I was planning on running across the country, I wanted it to mean more than just running across a country for self satisfaction and physical test. I wanted to make it bigger than myself, so I decided a charity needed to be involved in this run. I wanted to choose a charity that did not have much help, and wasn't well known. Right away, all the cancers were crossed off the list; they have a lot of help and are very well known.

About that time, I was looking for a place to live for my last semester of college because the lease for the current place I was living went from August to August and I didn't want to keep paying for rent on a place I wouldn't be living in for more than 4 months. Luckily, my mom had a friend who lived in Richmond. We met up with Jim for lunch one day to talk about possibly renting a room from him. During the course of the lunch he mentioned that his granddaughter wasn't doing too well. She had Juvenile Rumetoid Arthritis and some days she couldn't go to school. She had been hospitalized many times and she was only ten years old. I was in shock. I knew that elderly people got arthritis in their hands and knees and it was painful, but I never thought it got worse than them having trouble opening a jar. I didn't know it put people in the hospital, and I didn't know anyone under the age of 60 got the disease.

On the way home, I talked to my mom about it, and she told me that a few years back my cousin, Mia, had arthritis. Luckily it went into remission. This news was shocking so I went home and started researching arthritis in children.

I came across the Arthritis Foundation's website and right there on the front page it has pictures of people that reminded me of my grandparents. There were no pictures of little kids on there; I was a bit confused. The more I looked into it the more I was stunned. Seeing numbers like 300,000 kids afflicted and no cure in sight got me thinking.

Jim was involved with the Richmond, VA chapter of the Arthritis Foundation so I decided to ask him how I would go about raising money for them by running across the country. I guess he didn't see the question mark at the end of the email and I got an email back about how happy he was that I was going to do this for them. It's a good thing I had already decided to run for them, otherwise, I believe some disappointment would have been present. From there we discussed how to move forward with this, and make it all happen. That is when I decided on my monetary goal of $50,000 dollars. I thought it was a doable goal that would go a long way in terms of research for arthritis.

Talking to the Richmond chapter was a bit frustrating. It was not because they were not willing to help, and it wasn't because they were bad people. Everyone I met was extremely nice and very impressed that I had this idea. It was frustrating because they kept saying "if."

"If you do this . . ."

"If you make it . . ."

"If your body can take this . . ."

In reality, who could blame them? It was frustrating to think that someone doubted me, but I couldn't hold it against them. My story wasn't a very likely one.

Even though I wasn't getting a whole heap of help from the Arthritis Foundation at the time, I decided to move forward with the planning and work out a budget.

Being a college student, I was all for trying to save some money wherever I could; which is why I ran into some trouble with the budget.

Item	
Six pairs of Running Shoes	$570
Jogging stroller	$350.00
Food (approx $35/day)	$4,200
Lodging ($30/night)	$3,600
Incidentals (miscellaneous items, toiletries, etc. $15/week)	$255
Tent, sleeping bag, spare clothes, and rain gear	$325
Promotional Costs	$499
APPOXIMATE TOTAL	$ 9,999

I talked to my dad about it and since he is a Marine, he has the "plan for the worst and hope for the best" mentality. The problem with planning for the worst is that it means you're supposed to plan for the most expensive as well. $10,000 dollars was about $9,350 more than I had at the time. This wasn't good news but I still had all summer to work and to pick up extra shifts now and then.

First on the checklist was to finish school. I was so tired of school and I did not want to be there anymore. I had made up my mind in the fall of my junior semester that I would go to school non-stop until I graduated. That meant taking credits over Christmas break and a full semester over the summer so I could graduate a semester early. School during the summer, as well as work and now planning and training for this event was going to prove difficult.

I started looking into ways to raise the money. I had a job but it didn't pay very much and wouldn't be bringing in large sums of money. I was fortunate to still have the financial support from my parents as far as bills went. I did have to pay for gas but after I started looking at ways to get money, I decided maybe driving didn't need to happen. I had a bike and biked everywhere in the city from then on, unless I had to go onto the highway. Other ways I looked into money was selling the bike at the end of the semester. I sold all my CD's, older band t-shirts and I was able to sell more than I thought I could. Some people will buy anything.

I was still grossly under budget. I picked up as many shifts as I could and I did get some money for graduation, which helped more than I thought it might. But when I look back, I still left with way less money than I should've had. I left with about $2,000 in my bank account. I think my parents knew how far I was under budget but they didn't say anything. I decided not to tell anyone else because I didn't want their preconceived doubts to get deeper.

While planning for this trip we got a visit from my grandpa, Bob Muschek. He lives in Fullerton, California but was on the east coast for a business trip. During dinner I was told him about the trip and he told me about his recreational vehicle and how much he loves taking trips in it.

He has this little Chinook RV that is supposed to house two comfortably. In reality, I think that might be stretching it, but it says it sleeps two. He was asking me questions on how I was going to do certain sections of the country; mainly the desert and the mountains. I wasn't as concerned with these two areas as he was. For the desert, I thought would bring a couple gallons of water, a loaf of pb&j and be alright. After talking with one guy who had done this before, I found that the police and fire department are a possibility when it comes to help crossing the vastness of the desert's land. I'd notify the closest fire department of what I was doing and ask them if they would mind watching for vultures, just in case. The mountains I knew would be okay because I'm so comfortable there. That's the kind of running I love. The mountains relax me and I am so refreshed when I am there. Unfortunately, mere love for the mountains was not going to get me over them safely; especially in January. He was very concerned with both sections.

He mentioned that he was retiring soon and might be interested in driving some sort of support vehicle across the country but didn't make any promises at the time, and I didn't ask for any. The seed was planted in his head, and all I needed was time to let it grow.

A couple of weeks went by and every now and then I would get an email from my grandpa asking if I had come up with a way to get across the desert safely yet. Every time, I had to say no. It really hadn't come up because there were other things I had to worry about and it wasn't at the forefront of my concerns. The route was still in the works, I was still trying to find ways to fund the trip with corporate sponsors, fundraising had been turned on, and I had to figure out how to get the five pairs of shoes I needed to complete the trek. Those kinds of issues were more important to me at the time. The whole picture needed to be worked on instead of just focusing on a region of the country that was going to be a problem area. To him, I'm sure I sounded a bit unprepared, and to be honest, this might have worked to my benefit. After a couple emails going back and forth, he asked if he could drive the RV to support me. I did not turn it down. It was welcomed support. Why would I push the baby jogger any further than I had to?

On his next visit we sat down to figure out costs and how much my grandpa would drive. The gas for the RV and food for one more person were not budgeted into the original budget we had handed into the Arthritis Foundation. After discussing it, he decided that he would get me from California to the border of Texas; Post, Texas to be exact. After that he would return to his home in California and I would press on with the baby jogger. I knew that this was going to be an important support system because I had heard that the beginning of any long trip was the worst. I had talked to runners and bicyclists who had crossed the country and both said the same thing. The first week is the hardest. So to have a support crew in place for not only the first week, but the first month was incredible. Your body is getting used to the new punishment that it is not used to. Everything is terrible. Physically you feel like you're in hell and mentally, you can not fathom that you have to do this for x number of additional weeks. It turns into a mental trap that drags every part of you down. This support would help me finish.

When we sat down, we discussed cost. While driving 30 miles per day isn't a lot in terms of driving in an RV, the miles would add up between California and Texas. Unfortunately for us, miles mean gas, and gas means money. In the back of my mind I was a little bit nervous where the money was going to come from. We discussed who was going to pay for all of this and he took the ropes. He decided he would pay for the gas and food; for both of us while we were together. This was completely unexpected. I was expecting him to ask me to pay for at least my food. That would have been understandable.

This is when I started to think that people's generosity might play a more specific role in this run.

After I had talked to the Arthritis Foundation and was told that they do not help with funding efforts, but they did give some guidelines. They recommend not spending more than 30% of what you raise. I realized that this was going to be more complicated than just going door to door like I was selling Girl Scout cookies. So I turned to my dad—the man that coached my tee-ball teams.

When my dad jumped in to help me with all of the planning, we decided it would be best to set up a separate bank account for the fundraising efforts. This way, we would have control of when the money went in and what came out for costs without getting personal funds mixed up. Unfortunately, we couldn't have a joint account on something we were using for business purposes unless we had a small business license. So we got the small business license. Next, we went back to the bank and were able to get the account. The account's name was Patrick's Run 4 Arthritis, just like the website. We weren't sure where the $10,000 was going to come from. I obviously didn't have it and I was not going to ask my parents for that kind of money, they were already supporting me enough.

CHAPTER 4

No planning is without its bumps, bruises, and setbacks. I had my first potential setback at the end of the summer semester. Everyone I had talked to in the business department had told me that taking a full semester worth of credits was a bad idea for a summer schedule and that I was setting myself up to fail. After mid-terms in my finance class, I thought they had been right. Finance 311 at VCU is a horror story class. As a prerequisite to a class I needed to take next semester, I needed to pass. Otherwise, I would not graduate in December as planned. After speaking with the teacher I was reassured that I should see how the class plays out and keep trying. When the final came around I studied hard as usual and ended up passing that class. By how many points, I may never know, but I passed.

This was one more part of this trip that fell into place without explanation. One more reason, I was meant to go on this trip.

CHAPTER 5

I have to admit, I was not a strong public speaker. I wasn't scared of it; I just didn't believe myself to be good at it. Speaking to schools as a way of passing on the awareness of JRA was going to be the worst part of the trip. I was kind of dreading it. I didn't really see myself being able to keep a whole school interested in the reason I came to the school for very long.

I figured since I needed practice, I would need a "guinea pig" school. So, I chose a local school where I knew a lot of people. Saint Francis of Assisi Catholic School was my school for first and second grades and fifth through eighth grade. I still knew most of the teachers there and lots of the kids in my class who had younger siblings still in the school.

The first time I talked to the school, it was very awkward. I brought lots of props and thought of all the parts of the trip I could tell them about. I also told them about ultra marathons, and arthritis. I explained the different kinds of arthritis and how it was different from the arthritis that a lot of their grandparents may have had. Everything I was saying was in the future tense. It was hard to have everything seem like something I was going to do.

It sounds so big, it sounds unbelievable. It sounds like just a plan, and just something that is too big to comprehend even starting. Talking to schools during the run was much easier. There was even a big difference between the first and last school I spoke with and my comfort level. If anything, the trip gave me a boost on my public speaking skills.

CHAPTER 6

Training was a little bit difficult for me because the few months directly leading up to the run fell in my last semester of college. Along with the copious amounts of tests, papers, group projects, and studying that normally accompany the last semester of school I also had a part time job at my schools gym checking students and faculty into the building. I also had friends, and family and Katie who I wanted to spend time with. I was already in shape to run ultra marathons, but I didn't know how this run would differ from those; so I decided I would start from square one and pretend I wasn't in shape at all. I was not going to let myself slack on the training for this thing. I had to figure out how to train for high mileage without running the high mileage because of my time constraints.

The biggest obstacle while training was time. I sat down to go over my schedule and, except for weekends, I didn't have a single block of time where I had more than two hours to run. And that's not including the time it takes to shower after a run and travel time to my next engagement. I did, however, notice a bunch of smaller breaks in my schedule, sometimes three or four breaks of an hour or two. I figured I would use those and just run multiple times per day for shorter distances.

I'm not particularly fond of following someone else's training plan because everyone is different. There was no one in the world that had my exact schedule and was trying to do exactly what I was going to try to do. Besides scheduling differences, no one's body works exactly like mine does; be it muscular, skeletal, gastrointestinal, or mental. I am the only person that can find the training system that works best for me. There were several goals I had for my training plan.

1) I wanted to be strong. Not bulky, just strong. I wanted every muscle in my body to compliment my running. I would do this through pull ups, push ups, sit ups, and (as much as I hated it) weightlifting. I liked being outside more than inside, and many times, I would find a large rock (in the 35-50 lb range) while running on a trail and just stop and throw it around for a bit or run with it for a few yards. I also would climb trees while out in the woods, lift and throw logs, and just romp around the woods. It's amazing how many things that little kids do on a regular basis are still fun and can benefit your fitness level. I also ran barefoot and in Vibram Five Finger shoes a few runs per week to help strengthen all the little muscles in my feet.

2) I did not want to get injured. This one is easier said than done but I thought that if I played my cards right on the first goal, and was smart about the amount of running I was doing per day this would not be an issue. Besides, I was 21 and was Superman. Nothing could hurt me and I was invincible.

3) I wanted to be able to surprise myself on any given day of the week and run a marathon in under four hours. The timing issue came into play on this one but there were several nights that turned into rather late nights due to this goal.

4) I needed to get my recovery time down to an overnight process. This was done through constantly putting my body through intense exercises, yet eating enough calories to supply it with what it needs to repair itself. I thought that consistently pushing myself everyday with very few days off per month would help to achieve this.

A sample of one of my busiest days looked a little something like this:

4:30-5:30 am Wake up and bike to work

5:30-9:00 am Work

9:01-10:30 am Workout at the gym. Jump on the treadmill and run uphill for 15 minutes. Squats, leg extensions, hamstring curls, calf presses, push ups, pull ups, and sit ups in succession x2. Run on the Stairmaster for 10 minutes. Squats, leg extensions, hamstring curls, calf presses, push ups, pull ups, and sit ups in succession x2. Run outside as fast as I could for remaining time. I wanted to simulate running on legs that had been well used up, just like they would feel after running 30 or so miles the day before.

10:31-11:00 am Shower and bike to class

11:00 am—12:15 pm Class

12:15-12:29 pm Climb the stairs of whatever building I was in and try not to sweat

12:30-1:45 pm Class

1:45-2:00 pm Bike home to change

2:00-3:30 pm Run. Fast.

3:30-4:00 pm Shower and bike to class

4:00-6:40 pm Class

6:40-? Run, eat, and sleep

They were busy days, but I never got tired of it. The best part of my day was still to get outside and run around for awhile.

Another thing I did as training was to run ultra marathons on back to back weekends. This is somewhat uncommon except to the likes of those far superior to myself. I had set it up where I was going to try to do the 12 Hour Adventure trail run, the Great Eastern Endurance Run 100k and the Grindstone 100 mile run back to back to back.

There is a bit of background for the reason I chose these races as opposed to others.

In May of 2009 I had won the 24 hour Adventure trail run with 108 miles. This race was part of the Trail Runner Magazine's Trophy Series, which is a series where every race mile you complete counts as a point. If you place in the top three in a race you get added points. Having won the 24 hour race put me in the lead. After looking up the prizes for winning the whole Trophy Series, I discovered one of the prizes was an article in Trail Runner magazine, which is a nationally distributed magazine. I saw this as a great opportunity to expose the fundraising efforts of the cross country run.

From then on, the rest of the year's races were going to be Trophy Series races, except for the Grindstone 100. I wanted to do that one because it claimed to be the "hardest 100 miler this side of the 100th meridian."

I signed up for the Burning River 100 in August, the 12 Hour Adventure Trail Run in September, and the Great Eastern Endurance Run 100k. I knew I had a decent chance of at least placing in the 12 Hour race because it was a smaller race at the time and had a much smaller field.

My strategy all summer and fall was to train hard for the races while running more on roads to try to get my feet and bones ready for the hard pavement I would encounter on the cross country run. As far as the race strategy, I would run fast in the 12 hour to try to win and get the added points; plus, the number of miles was up to me, so every mile I completed counted as one more point. My plan for the 100k was simply to finish. The field was much more competitive in that race and it was in the mountains, boasting more than 15,000 feet of elevation change throughout the 100 kilometers. I would use all the time they allowed for the race and just remain relaxed so I would complete the race, get the points, and still not wreck myself going into the Grindstone 100.

The 12 hour went as planned. I ran hard, accomplished my goal of placing first with 71.5 miles; even though the two hours following the race were taken up by throwing up everything I had eaten that day and more all because I got a little bit competitive with the relay teams that were running the same course as the solo runners. Knowing that I beat the relay teams totals for the day helped ease some of the pain of barfing.

The Great Eastern Endurance Run did not go as planned. The weather was not very agreeable that day and this caused many people to drop out. I was running comfortably, smooth and without any problems. At around the halfway point aid station I was told I was in third place. This was fantastic, except my competitive side came out and I started running harder and faster. I caught the current second place runner which now put me in second place. I couldn't stand the thought of losing that spot and so I continued to run hard despite the cold rain that the weather so conveniently dealt us. The first place runner was more than an hour ahead of me so there was no catching that speed demon but at the end of the race I secured the 2nd place spot, earning me more points than I had anticipated earning toward the Trophy Series. Earning more points was the good news; the bad news was that I hadn't stuck to the plan. Running hard put an added stress on all my muscles and mentality. Running hard up and down mountains had given me a slight pain in my right foot that was with me until the end of the race. But coming in second place put me on this strange cloud 9 that made me feel invincible.

The week leading up to Grindstone I took it easy as I did the previous week and did some light running and walking, but mostly I rested in somewhat fearful anticipation of the upcoming race. I also iced the foot that was hurting me, and babied it in hopes that it would heal fully in a week. I didn't know what was exactly wrong with it. All I knew was it hurt.

Grindstone starts at 6 pm on a Friday and the cutoff time is 38 hours later on Sunday at 8 am. Running up and down more mountains in the dark on the winding single track did a number on my mental state for the run. I was also pushing harder than I should have. When I got to the aid station at mile 37 we were weighed in. I was down 6 lbs. Having lost 6 pounds in the first half of the race meant that I was not keeping up with my nutrition the way I needed to be. Hearing this was the final straw to my frustration and I dropped out of the race. My muscles were way more tired than they should have been at mile 37 and my foot was giving me trouble from the start. The decision to drop out of that race was incredibly difficult but it taught me an invaluable lesson: I am not invincible.

My dad was at Grindstone with me and when I decided to drop he was the one to drive me back to the start of the race where my car was and where my friend/pacer, Adam, was asleep in the tent. On the drive back we were talking about dropping and how it would help me in the long run. It not only taught me that I wasn't invincible, it taught me what it felt like to quit something. I hated that. It was a terrible feeling and I hoped I'd never feel it again. I was able to think of the long road across the country and how this experience would give me a new perspective on what it means to be mentally, more than physically, tough. I would remember Grindstone and the big DNF (Did Not Finish) letters that stood next to my name in the final standings many times during the cross country run. The other big lesson I got from Grindstone was the importance of sticking to my plans. I had done my homework and figured out what I needed to do to finish all three races on back to back to back weekends.

CHAPTER 7

By this point, my dad had taken on a second job helping me with the logistics for the trip. He was the one to make the website and helped me figure out how to handle the money for the fundraising without breaking any laws. Once we opened the website, we started getting donations, sometimes very large donations. People were being very supportive of the trip. They would write little encouraging notes and urge me to keep going no matter what because they knew I could do it. I had people I didn't even know thanking me for doing this for the kids with arthritis before I had even started. This was great because it put a little bit more emphasis on why I was doing this yet it added a lot of pressure as well.

Back in May when I won the 24 Hour race, I was very excited and wrote an email to my Uncle Bob, a very fast marathoner, telling him about the race. In it, I also mentioned that I was thinking about running across the country. I got a call that evening from my uncle and at the end, my Aunt Vickie got on the phone. She expressed special interest in the part about me running across the country. I told her at the time I wasn't certain on anything but would keep her up to date. Fast forward a bit and after informing her about doing it as a fundraiser she was 150% in. She jumped on board and started contacting people; everyone she could think of that had anything to do with either running or arthritis. Every time I talked to her it seemed she had some piece of news that was incredibly helpful. She had worked out a whole big send-off on the California end which would be at Bella Terra Mall. The local chapter of the Arthritis Foundation, which is led by Amy Daugherty, was helping to make the send off a large event. Emails were flying back and forth by the minute and every day the list of people who were involved grew. Right from the start, I had an incredible support team.

CHAPTER 8

When I woke up on December 2, 2009 I had an eerie feeling. I woke up thinking, "One month from today I'll be in California and I'll start running east." Time with family, friends, and especially Katie was highly valued at this point. I was getting closer and closer everyday to leaving everything I was familiar with for a planned four months but it could have been a lot longer for all I knew. There were so many unknowns, so many variables, and so many things that could go wrong. Katie and I went to schools that were an hour and a half apart, so we were used to only spending one day per week together, but as the trip got closer, the time was more and more important.

It was a mad dash for the 2nd of January and time wasn't slowing down. It constantly felt like there was so much to do and so much to get ready for. Little by little, things fell into place and the trip was planned. I had written to several companies looking for sponsorship for the trip, and kept getting overly polite emails back from the companies stating that they would not be able to sponsor me. Though, I did get two emails back from two different companies that said quite the opposite. SmartWool Socks and Gu energy gel both decided that I was worth the risk and they decided that I'd be worth sponsoring. One of the heads of the research and developing for SmartWool, Zach, contacted me and asked if he could send me some socks that I could beat up and wear over the course of the trip and give him feedback on. I agreed and so became a sock tester.

Planning was falling into place, my jogger and most of my equipment was shipped to California and I had trained. I was in the best shape of my life, yet part of me felt like there was no way I could prepare for this endeavor completely. Mentally I was both confident in my abilities, and incredibly nervous. I couldn't quite put my finger on what scared me most about the trip; all I knew was as time grew closer I became more terrified. It was a fear of the vast unknown, of what would happen in the four months I had planned for the trip. I didn't know what I would see, I didn't know who I'd meet, what experiences I'd have or how my body would react to that much road running.

I had to downplay my fear simply because I think Katie and my mom were already nervous enough. Expressing my nervousness would have only made them even more scared.

December 12th I graduated from Virginia Commonwealth University with a Bachelors of Science Degree in Business Marketing. I'm not big on parties but my mom insisted on having a graduation party to double as a going away party. So, I agreed. As I looked around the gathering of people, I was having second thoughts about the trip. All of these people were there to support me graduating and to see me before I left on my big endeavor. I couldn't let them down.

Chapter 9

December 26 was the day I finished packing and drove up to Katie's parent's house in Arlington. It's only 5 minutes from the airport so it only made sense to stay there for the night and have them give Katie and I a ride to the airport the next day.

I hugged my mom goodbye at the house. I didn't really want her to drive me up because I didn't want her to cry. I'm not very good at seeing people cry without crying myself; so I thought I'd eliminate any chance of waterworks. My dad drove me up to Katie's house and we had a talk. It wasn't the kind of talk where I could tell I was in trouble or just small talk or even the standard parental saying of "we'll love you whether you finish or not." He had backpacked through Europe when he was my age and I'll never forget what he told me. He looked at me and said, "Follow your gut. You're a smart kid, and you know when things aren't right. Listen to the little voice that tells you when things aren't the way they should be." And that was that.

On December 27, 2009 I flew out of National Airport with Katie on our way to Montana. We were going to go to her friends' Sara and Josh Louk's wedding on the 28th. Then, on the 30th, we'd fly to San Diego to visit my Uncle Bob, Aunt Vickie, and cousins Maddy, Mandy, and baby Bobby and stay for New Year's Eve. On New Year's Day, we'd take the train from San Diego to Fullerton, where my grandfather lived. He would pick us up from the train station and drive Katie and myself down to Huntington Beach where I would touch the water and run 5 miles to Bella Terra Mall, where the big celebration would take place on January 2nd: my official start date.

I was especially glad I got to spend a couple of days with just Katie. My relationship with her is a bit different. We were good friends in high school but only started dating in college. We had a long distance relationship but since we skipped the whole "awkward getting to know who the other person is" part of the dating game, it seemed to work. I knew I was going to miss her a lot. A week is a while when you want to see someone every day but four months sounds like years when you're used to thinking in terms of weekends.

Montana was beautiful state. Had I been running the northern route, I would have liked to run through the whole thing. The wedding was very nice and quaint. It was completely snow covered outside and gave everything a very fresh feeling. Everyone had a good time but before we knew it, it was time to leave the chilly—6 degrees Fahrenheit in Montana for the mid 70s of California.

When traveling, everything seems longer when you're anticipating something big. For some reason, I didn't want that night time plane ride to end. I was sitting next to Katie, her hand securely in mine, looking out our little window at the vast, dark, land below and the stars still higher than our plane. Looking over a giant mass of land is not the best way to spend your time when you're about to take on something like running the span of something that takes more than 6 hours to fly across.

After reaching the San Diego airport and meeting up with my Uncle Bob, we went back to his house where I stayed in my cousin Maddy's room and fell asleep staring at her pink painted walls.

The next day, New Year's Eve, we caught up with the relatives and went to the San Diego Zoo. Doing regular vacation-like things were good because it gave me time to relax and try not to think about the trip so much. My cousins Maddy, Mandy, and baby Bobby had more energy than I could have possibly imagined. Not a bad kind of energy, but the kind that would give the Energizer Bunny a run for his money. That night my Aunt Vickie's family came over for a cookout and to visit with us. Being that they had little kids, they left as the Ball dropped on Time Square . . . on New York's time. That left Katie and I time to (try to) stay up to watch it on California's time. Traveling on planes tends to suck the energy right out of me so I'm sure I dozed off a few times, but I did see the Ball drop and was able to wish her a happy new year.

New Years Day brought with it a train ride up the coast from San Diego to Los Angeles. The train ride was great, we were able to see the Pacific Ocean for pretty much the whole way; but it didn't last long enough. I was really getting scared at this point. Doubts were flying in and out of my head faster than I could comprehend what was going on. A couple of times I actually got dizzy and just closed my eyes to try and relax for a bit.

Before I left Virginia, my mom gave me a little spiral notebook to write in as I traveled. I thought the train would be a good time to write the first entry. It went a little something like this:

"It's the day before the actual big sendoff. On the train ride up from Sand Diego I was on the verge of tears the whole way. I held Katie's hand the entire ride and was not ready to get off the train. There is something weird going on with my lungs."

That last part about the lungs made me even more nervous. I'm very allergic to cats. My Uncle and Aunt have a cat but while I was there he stayed in the garage; unfortunately, his dander stayed in my lungs. The real problem was that the longer I stay in a house with cats, the longer it takes for the dander to get out of my lungs, so I still was wheezing even though I wasn't in the house anymore.

My grandfather met us at the train station and picked us up, and we were supposed to drive straight to Huntington Beach where I would touch the water and run 5 miles to Bella Terra Mall. He suggested we go back to his house for lunch first. Little did I know, he was stalling.

After grabbing a quick sandwich back at his house we made our way down to Huntington Beach. We pulled into the parking lot and ahead of us was the Pacific Ocean. Then he pointed just off to the right and said, "Hey, we know them!" I looked out my window and saw my parents! They had flown out last minute to surprise me at the start. Katie and I both threw open the doors and ran to them. Trying to hold in tears for a couple days now was useless. I cried. I couldn't believe they had come all the way out for it.

"We never missed a tee-ball game. How were we going to miss something this big?"

We all walked down and I put my hands in the frigid Pacific Ocean. I looked out at the ocean and around at all the people who happened to be at the beach that day. I looked again out over the huge body of water, turned around and started running. That day was only five miles and yet my lungs hurt so badly. I couldn't seem to suck in enough air to keep my lungs satisfied. The first mile was agonizing. The second was terrible. The third I cursed the existence of cats. The fourth I wondered if all 2,553 miles would be like this. And the fifth I was very happy to be done.

My mom and dad met in Southern California and still had friends there so that night we all went to their friend's Margaret and Bob's house for dinner. I had met them several times and always have fun with them. Bob's a coke dealer! I just get a kick out of saying that. Actually, coke is petroleum by product, and he sells it. It's not the white powdery stuff that comes to mind, but he sure enjoys telling people he's a coke dealer.

We had a meal fit for kings. It was my first pre-run meal and was absolutely delicious. Looking back on the amount of food I ate, and the number of houses I ate at, I could put a cookbook together of all the delicious dishes I had that I hadn't had before. Many of them were old family recipes that they made especially for me from families all in the southern half of this country.

We stayed at my grandpa's house that night. And Katie and I stayed up late talking. This would be the last time I got to see her and only her before she flew back to Virginia the following night. I did not want that night to end. Minutes seemed to act more like seconds. And seconds flew by like a blur. I would have given anything just to be able to slow time down for awhile. I was scared and didn't sleep much that night.

CHAPTER 10

January 2nd, 2010 was the big day. I awoke after a couple hours of sleep with a stomach ache. Not the kind you get when you have the flu or when you eat something strange. It was the "butterflies" kind of stomach ache. I quickly packed up my stuff into my backpacking backpack, ate half of a banana and was out the door. We drove down to Bella Terra Mall where the ceremony would take place. There was a bearded runner already there. He looked young and had on brightly colored shorts and a running hat on. He asked if I was Patrick and I assured him I was. He then proceeded to pull out a local newspaper article and ask for my autograph. I had never in my life been asked for my autograph, so I wrote my name next to the article. Gus, as I found out his name later, had come out to run with me on my first day. He was a really funny guy and quite the tour guide as well. He knew the area we were running through very well and gave all the people who were running with us nice little pieces of information all day.

As we were standing around my grandfather's RV, more and more people started showing up. I was a little bit surprised since I didn't expect too many people to come. But then again, my Aunt Vickie had put this together so it was well organized. I met people who I had only met through an email. I met kids with arthritis and the amazing parents who take care of them. They were all thanking me and telling me how great it was to have someone do something for their kid. Meeting those parents and kids was turning out to be much more emotional than I expected it to be.

When we went into the center of the out-door mall there were TV cameras set up, and a podium, and a marching band. That's right, a marching band. I made my way around to all the people who were already there and thanked them for coming. I talked to people from the local Arthritis Foundation chapter, and the families they supported. I talked to local runners and some friends of my parents from when they lived in California. It seemed like the amount of people to talk to was growing faster than I was capable of keeping up with. But before I knew it, it was time to start the pre-run ceremony.

I sat down with the head of the Arthritis Foundation, Amy, the Mayor Pro-Tem, Jill, and an eleven year old girl, Mikayla. We each had something to say. First the Mayor Pro-Tem spoke and said some very nice things about me. I had a little bit of a hard time soaking it all in because I hadn't done it yet. This was just the beginning. They had no idea what would happen. I had no idea what would happen. For all any of us knew I could've been hit by a bus the very first day! And these were the kinds of things that were running through my head.

Next on the microphone was Amy. She was very good at informing people about the Arthritis Foundation and all the ways they can help kids with arthritis. It was nice to have someone there who really knew what they were talking about and could inform people about the disease from a professional point of view. I had done my homework and I could repeat some statistics, but I wasn't quite the same as someone who did that as their job. Then she introduced Mikayla.

In the past, Mikayla had spoken to Congress begging them for Arthritis research funding. The girl has got her public speaking credentials and isn't even a teenager yet. I knew she would say something that day but I wasn't at all ready for what she hit me with.

I've been called a lot of names in my day. Mostly goofy ones that apply to a dumb haircut I had in high school or words that mean 'doofus' that were made up by my brother, Kevin, on the spot right before we started an epic battle of wrestling wars in the house only to be kicked out of the house shortly afterwards by my mother for being "too big for that." I was expecting something along the lines of, "Thank you Patrick, it's really cool what you're going to try to do." Instead she started citing the definition of a hero and what it means to her, and how the run related to her and her definition of a hero. A hero? She sort of blindsided me with it but she gave me a rubber bracelet that says, "Kids get arthritis too." It's white with blue words but I found out it's actually blue with white painting on it because I haven't taken it off since the start, and the white paint is starting to come off. When it was my turn to talk, I forgot everything that I had preplanned. I just made it up. I was mostly surprised at how emotional the start was becoming. But then I glanced in the back row and I saw both my parents crying, and half the audience crying and so I decided to cut it short and start the thing.

I walked my packed baby jogger up the side of the crowd and made my way to the "official starting line." Then my cousins, Maddy and Mandy held out a giant paper starting line and said "GO!"

It didn't tear because I wasn't running fast enough. I'm not sure if you've ever tried to break a giant piece of paper by just running into it, but it's hard; so I threw it over my head and made my way to the street with Gus, my Uncle Bob, and several kids, including Mikayla. Gus looked at Mikayla and said, "Hey! You're running pretty good, are you sure you have arthritis?"

She replied with, "Yea, I'm sure, I had joint injections yesterday so I could run today."

That hit me right in the heart.

This was the big moment. Starting here was what I had trained for, planned for, and looked forward to for so many months. In one thought, it felt like I was literally running away from my family and friends. But it also felt like I was running toward all of them and toward the long road that would take me to them. Leaving the starting line, I was already looking forward to seeing them on the other side of the country.

By the time we got across the parking lot and onto the street, the kids had turned back and it was just my uncle, Gus, and me. It was a warm day already and it was only going to get warmer.

We got about 4 miles down the road and my parents and Katie were there with an aid station. They had cookies, and bananas, and water. It was perfect, but it was a luxury I tried not to get accustomed to because this would be the only day I would have this. Unfortunately, I was now feeling a little sick and didn't feel much like eating. I think it was a combination of not sleeping well the night before, all the excitement of the morning, and knowing that in a couple hours I would have to say goodbye to Katie for quite awhile. As the day wore on I was feeling worse and worse. I was sluggish and slow and I still couldn't seem to breathe right. It was very frustrating for many reasons but mainly because I knew that it was just a rough day but it was the first day, it was supposed to be the easiest. I was fresh, had zero miles on my legs and was supposed to feel on top of the world. Also, I was running with people and I'm sure they were having second thoughts about my abilities after seeing me that first day.

Later in the day, as it got hotter, Gus took off his shirt and revealed one tattoo on each of his shoulders. The left shoulder said, "Badwater (Lowest point)" and the right shoulder said, "Mt. Whitney (highest point)." I knew that could only mean one thing. Gus had run the Badwater Ultra marathon. 135 miles starting in Badwater, the lowest point in the continental United States at 282 feet below sea level, and ending at the portals of Mt. Whitney, the highest point in the continental United States. The tough part about the race isn't the distance; it's the heat. The race is run in July. Temperatures can get up to 130 degrees Fahrenheit. This race has always been a dream of mine to run, and to meet someone who had done it? Now I was the one who wanted the autograph. I asked Gus about the tattoo, confirming my assumption.

"So, Gus. You've run Badwater?"
"Yea, a couple of my friends and I ran it on our own a couple of years ago. We had a support vehicle, but we all ran basically our own pace."

About halfway through the day, a friend from high school, Keaton, came out to run with me. He also brought his friend. Keaton was living in the area at the time, and wanted to come out and run the first day with me. In all the starting line excitement I accidentally told him I was starting at the wrong place, but somehow he figured out how to find us.

Toward the end of the run I realized the main reason I felt so crummy, I hadn't eaten anything except a half of a banana all day. It was a dumb mistake and I was frustrated I had made such a stupid mistake on the first day, but I started eating and my legs and energy levels started flowing a little better. The first day ended at Brea Mall and was welcomed so I could sit next to Katie and spend as much time as I could with her and my parents between now and when they would have to fly out that night.

CHAPTER 11

Somewhere along the flying emails and different people who were thrown into the mix were Kim and Walter. Walter had arthritis himself and has had more surgeries than I could count. When they heard that I was starting near them they immediately invited me to stay the first night at their house. As if that wasn't enough, they offered to throw a fundraiser pasta party.

When we all showed up I couldn't believe the amount of people that were there. I immediately started meeting people but realized my skills for remembering names were severely lacking. Names went in one ear and out the other. I couldn't understand why I couldn't remember anyone's name. Regardless of current skill level for remembering names, there were a ton of people there. All the kids were in the back yard inside a moon bounce. Had no one been watching, I might have been in there too.

There were multiple types of pasta and multiple sauces! It was a smorgasbord of food—buffet style—my favorite. Everything food-wise was delicious. Everyone was incredibly welcoming and kind. We all ate our fills, and then some. I could not have planned the close of the first day to go any better; yet in the back of my mind I knew that I would be saying goodbye to my parents (again) and Katie in only a few hours. It left a sour taste in my mouth just thinking about it. So I distracted myself with talking to people; something I'm not usually too good at.

After a few very quick hours, the time came for Katie to leave with Bob and Vickie, Maddy, Mandy and Baby Bobby. My parents thought it'd be a good idea to get all the goodbyes over with at once so they left at the same time. I walked them all out to their cars hugged and kissed them all and that was it. Seeing their cars drive away was incredibly difficult and a feeling of loneliness flooded me all at once. It was a feeling I would experience many times on this trip.

After they left I got very tired and decided it was a good idea to go to sleep. That night I lay in bed and stared at the pink and purple walls of Walter and Kim's daughter's room, where I was staying. It was my first night staying in a house where people invited me into their home as a complete stranger. It was comforting but at the same time, the thought of four more months still scared me.

CHAPTER 12

Day two brought with it more incredibly nice weather. Meeting at the same place I had ended the previous day I met a little girl named Caitlyn. She was a bit shy but a very cute little blonde girl who had arthritis. Her and her family had come back early from their family vacation to come meet me. I couldn't believe their support and devotion to the cause. After talking with them for awhile, Caitlyn gave me a baseball card with her picture on it. She played sports even though she had arthritis. I thanked them all for coming and thanked Caitlyn for the card as I tucked it into my pack.

It was cool in the morning but didn't stay that way for long. I had company for awhile and that was very nice. Kim, her friend Susan, and their trainer Tom all started off the day with me. Unfortunately, Susan got sick in the beginning so she didn't stay too long.

As we started up some long climbs of the valleys it got incredibly windy. The canyons seemed to form wind tunnels that forced the wind directly into us. Kim decided to call it a day after about an hour and it was her longest run so far. Since then, she has run several half marathons!

Tom stuck around for awhile. He stayed with me into the heat of the day and ran further than he ever had before. Tom was Susan and Kim's trainer and was built like a freight train. He was stocky and looked like he played football. He looked to be around my age, but he had a pretty legitimate job as a personal trainer so after much of the morning, I finally asked him how old he was.

"I'm 20, but I'll be 21 next month." He stated.

I asked him if he was getting crazy on his birthday.

"With any luck I will. A bunch of friends and I are going to Las Vegas for my party."

Now that's a bash he won't forget . . . or will he?

After some long climbing and some long descents, he called it a day. From then on I was on my own. After a couple wrong turns, running out of water, some dry heat I wasn't quite acclimated to, and a stop by a convenience store for a slushee, I made it to the end of my second day in time to meet up with Kim, Walter, and Catherine. I said my goodbyes to Kim and Walter and said my hellos to Catherine.

Catherine was the head of the Arthritis Foundation for Redlands, CA. Immediately she showed me nothing but kindness and offered me something to eat. I had packed a couple of extra peanut butter and jelly's and started going to town on those. I wasn't sure the exact mileage of the day but it took me a long time and I was tired. Catherine was a mother of 7 grown kids so she had a very motherly air about her. She drove me all around Loma Linda and gave me a little tour along with some history about the place. She then took me to the family's house I would be staying with the next three days. Yes, three days. They heard about the run and offered to take me all three days I would be in the area. Talk about hospitality. I stayed with Charles, Linda, and their two kids Charlie and Julia. Julia had arthritis herself but it didn't slow her down. She still was a normal kid and swam quite a bit. Charlie, their son, was really funny. He was incredibly smart and has won several academic awards since I met him. Linda had a very different sense of humor but I seemed to get along with her just fine. Charles was a hulking mammoth of a man and a cyclist. I think he was rather modest about how good he was at it, but I got the feeling he was quite good because there were several pictures of him riding and every picture looked like a blur. Charles was also very familiar with the area; which was a good thing for me because he knew a good trail I could take to avoid being on the roads all day for the next day.

Chapter 13

I took Charles' advice and took the trail he told me about for my third day's run. Since this one didn't have roots and rocks jutting up every couple of feet, or trees surrounding it, it wasn't quite the kind of trail I was used to. It was paved but it was made for biking so I didn't have any problems with cars on it. I remained on the trail for the majority of the day but had to get back to the roads for the last 10 miles. The trail was nice and quiet and I had no troubles with it. When I got back to the roads I had forgotten how loud traffic could be.

I was running along and all of a sudden, something hit me like a semi-truck. It was something I had never experienced and I thought I might be sick. It was hunger; but not just ordinary hunger. This hunger struck with a vengeance. I had been eating every half hour or so and piled on the food after the run and at dinner; but apparently, all the calorie burning had caught up to me. Luckily I was across the street from a pizza place when I realized what I needed. I went inside and ordered a large supreme pizza. Waiting the 10 minutes for the pizza seemed to be the longest 10 minutes of my life. I was sitting on the bench outside. I could feel my life force getting sucked out of me by the second. When the lady inside waved to me signaling it was done I went to stand up and couldn't. I had to lean over sideways, and use the momentum to get onto my arms and do a push-up and squat together to propel myself up. It was the most awkward way to get up. When I got inside the lady asked me if I was okay. I said, "I'm fine, just a little hungry," received the pizza, and started walking down the street. I had to meet Catherine in just a little while and I didn't know how much further I had to go so I decided I'd move and eat to save some time. The pizza was so loaded I had to eat it backwards crust first and just slide it into my mouth. One slice in I could already feel my battery starting to recharge, so I moved a little faster. Two slices down and I was feeling good; yet still hungry. I kept eating and every piece gave me more and more energy.

After 7 slices I was full; but I didn't know what I'd do with the last slice so I tucked the box under my arm and started running down the street. It was an awesome feeling to get full and feel smooth running again. I came across a homeless guy and offered him my last piece of pizza. The only way I knew he was homeless was because he had a sign, "I AM HOMELESS. GIVE ME MONEY."

I showed him the box with the pizza inside and said, "You want a piece of pizza? It's supreme . . ."

"Nah, man, you got any money? I need money." The older man replied.

"Sorry, I just have pizza. Good luck."

"Whatever, man."

I kept running and after ten minutes my stomach told me it was ready for the last slice. I ate it, disposed of the box and picked up the pace. I figured that if 8 slices could keep me fueled for another 40 minutes, I'd make it to meet Catherine with no problem. About half an hour later the crippling hunger was back. Luckily, I was close enough to make it to the end without any negative side effects.

When Catherine picked me up I was about ready to just roll myself into the car and take a nap, but she had other plans. She knew of a rheumatologist in the area and asked if I wanted to meet her. Seeing as I was doing this for arthritis and had never talked to an actual doctor to learn all I could about it, I figured it was a good idea. Luckily, she let me take a shower before we went. On the way there my stomach was really hurting from being so hungry but I had already eaten all that I had packed for immediately after the run. I couldn't believe I was this hungry. The amount of food I would need and being this hungry were parts of the run I hadn't taken much into account.

Luckily, just before the rheumatologist there was an In-and-Out Burger, a fine West Coast cuisine. Catherine asked if I was hungry and I could not turn it down; especially being In-and-Out. I don't normally eat too much fast food, but I'll make an exception for In-and-Out. Maybe it's because I'm only in California once every couple of years, and maybe it's because it really does taste that good. When I chomped down on my Double Double, and half the ingredients came oozing out of the bun and the lettuce and tomato slid part-way out the back, I knew it was because it really did taste that good. I was energized again and could keep running if I had to. I was glad I didn't have to, but I could've.

Unfortunately for us, the rheumatologist was not working the day we went by so I didn't get to meet her.

That night, we discussed the next day's events. There would be a news story to be taped at around 2 o'clock on Juvenile Arthritis and they wanted me there for it. I was happy to do the interview except it was about an hour's drive away. I also had to run 31 miles. Having the two events going on the same day, and one of them requiring around 5 hours means having to run a lot faster than normal or start earlier. So I opted to start early.

CHAPTER 14

Day four started, of course, at the exact spot I ended day three. The morning air was very chilly so I waited in Linda's car for the reporter who was coming for a newspaper article. When he came, we shared a few words, answered a few questions and he tried to take a picture. From what I hear, it didn't turn out because it was still dark.

I started off down the road with my headlamp and reflective belt on and all I saw was a 6 foot circle of pavement in front of me. It was incredibly peaceful. The first couple miles were very difficult for me because my legs were not working as smoothly as they had been the past three days. I could tell I had put many miles on them already and this was the point where the actual running portion of the trip became a bit difficult.

I had many turns to take today, but I wouldn't have to worry about those for awhile. I was enjoying being outside and doing exactly what I was supposed to be doing. As I made my way down the road while it was still dark the only thing to interrupt the quiet of the morning was my breathing and the slight tapping of my shoes on the white line of the road. They formed a rhythm you can't find during any other time of day or in any other aspect of life. It was a beat that put me into a state of mind I often find if I'm running in the mountains with no one around for miles. It was a trance-like state of mind and everything left my brain. I didn't have to think about running, it just happened and everything was at peace.

As the sun began to slightly illuminate the scenery around me in a pink and orange glow I realized the true beauty of what I was looking at. It looked nothing like what I had around my home or anywhere on the East Coast for that matter. There were large hills all around but they were mostly barren with only a few brown scraggily trees on them. The hills gave the effect that I was in a canyon and on the far side, the road made its way out of it. They were a texture that you can't find on the east coast because all of our hills have vegetation to hide the bumps and changes in topography. I started to think about what caused the little ridges and why the part I was running on was a valley. I hoped it was a result of a river a million years ago and not caused by people messing up the beauty that nature clearly had a better eye for. A few of the hills had some small patches of tall brown grass that swayed in the chilly morning's wind. If a stronger breeze blew I would try to quiet my breathing so I could hear the large blades of grass shift in the winds. I got good at it and learned to quiet everything to the point where the only proof I was still breathing was the fact that you could see it.

I was running straight into the sunrise and the scenery changed between the hills and orange groves. When I finally remembered I was running I had to check my phone to make sure I hadn't missed any turns. When I clicked it on, I realized that I had been running for over two hours and couldn't remember a single step of it. If you asked me about the scenery though, I could tell you about every blade of grass and every sound I heard.

Luckily, I hadn't missed any turns. However, I was about a tenth of a mile away from my first one. This brought me into and out of neighborhoods buried into the side of hills and even though the houses interrupted the view of the hills, it really didn't bother me.

I kept on rolling until the last part of the run. I had run out of secondary roads and needed to find my own way to get down a 13 mile stretch of I-10 because, technically, it is illegal to run on the interstates.

When I got to the intersection of I-10, I found my answer: a trail. I think at one point it was a road because it was the same width as a single lane road but it was all I needed. I started running on it but realized that I had to do 13 miles in an hour in order to finish at the time that I was going to be picked up by Linda to drive up to the interview. That just wasn't going to happen. The American record for the half marathon is 59:43 set by Ryan Hall. For starters, I'm no Ryan Hall, and to finish it off, my legs were in no order to go that fast; but I could try. I tried to pick up the pace and hold it but it was just too hard. It felt like my already inflexible legs were tighter than usual and making them flex and stretch at a faster pace felt like being put through medieval torture. I would have to settle for my best. Unfortunately, my best was put to the test against a very windy section between hills. So much so that there were windmills all around. Hundreds. They were on the flat valley floor, and all the way up the sides of the hills and on top. It was the biggest windmill farm I had ever seen.

When Linda picked me up I was 4 miles shy of my stopping point. It was frustrating to be in pain and to need to go fast and not be able to. It was frustrating to not be able to finish what I had planned on doing. And it was frustrating to feel like I was already behind on the fourth day. It was too early to fall behind and I didn't want to get behind on mileage in the first week. I was overall cranky and upset but would have to put that aside for the interview.

It was nice to get to know Julia on the way up to the interview. She was a cute seven year old girl who had a strange love for the band Abba. We listened to the band she loved the entire time we drove.

The interview went well, and I think I was more nervous about it than Julia was. She was very well spoken and knew more than I thought she would for her age about arthritis. Julia explained how her joint pain affected her daily, and how she had to deal with it constantly.

"I just try to not pay attention to it too much when I'm playing." She stated simply. She sounded so much older than her age. The interviewer's expressions changed dramatically from a sort of happy interested to shocked and horrified when she went from talking to me to Julia. I had heard many kids talk about what they go through on a daily basis dealing with their disease but it never got any easier to hear. The initial punch of hearing a kid talk about how much pain they were in at any given time never got easier to take. I could tell by the look on her face, that this would be one interview that the news anchor wouldn't forget; and it had nothing to do with me.

CHAPTER 15

That night we, again, made plans for the next day. This time, my grandfather, Bob, would be picking me up and I would be saying goodbye to the family I had gotten to know so well over the past three days. I had families to stay with the next two nights and then I'd be in the desert and my grandfather would take the helm of his RV and we would be on the road together for the next month.

All that evening I was in pain. My legs hurt, my feet hurt, my ankles, bones, hips, back, shoulders, neck, and my pride hurt. I hadn't finished the day's miles and I knew I had to add them onto tomorrow and tomorrow I had to do a lot of climbing. I was going to be running up to the high desert of Joshua Tree, CA and I didn't really know what to expect. All I knew was that I was dreading the next day. When I called Katie that night I told her I didn't know if I could finish. Frustration was taking over and I was exhausted and in pain and I could not fathom doing this for another 100 or so days. She helped remind me that it's *only running* and it's what I do. I didn't need to think about next week or even two days from now. I just needed to take one day at a time, and when that was too much to think about just take it one step at a time.

I have to admit, I didn't believe her at the time, but before I went to sleep that night I told myself I only had to get through tomorrow. Surprisingly, the next morning when I woke up, I only thought about that day. I felt refreshed and new. My legs weren't as sore and nothing above my waist hurt at all. I told myself it would be a good day and I only had to make it as far as I wanted. I didn't even need to finish the day's miles. Who cared if this thing took a year? Not me, I was going to stay optimistic.

My grandpa picked me up and we drove to where I left off. When I started running I felt that the freshness in my legs and body were only a trick my body played on me to get me out the door. My legs were very sore and my ankles were killing me, but as I kept running, more blood flowed and it became much easier. I got to the end of the little road I was on and reached the end of road I was legally allowed to run on. I had to run on I-10 for 4 miles. I had heard of people getting kicked off the highway and put in the back of the police car so they could drive you to the next exit. I didn't want to do that because that would mean once I got to the end of the trip I would have run across the whole country without running that 4 mile section. So I booked it. I knew this because a square box in the sky opened up and called my number.

Grandpa leapfrogged with me every half mile or so just in case the 5-0 gave me any issues. He drove forward and pulled over on the shoulder to wait for me to pass and then he'd drive forward again. I tried to just relax, roll, and run as fast as I could. I was so appreciative of Grandpa for leapfrogging on the highway. It was a security blanket of someone in the region who could back up my story of cross country running if I ran into issues. It was also nice to know that if a semi-truck squashed my brains all over the pavement that someone I knew was going to be able to explain why I was running where I was.

As I got off the highway and got onto the road that would take me straight up to the high desert Grandpa stopped again. This time he had water and snacks for me. He was ready for full support and it gave me something to look forward to every couple miles for the rest of the day. There was a very long and straight stretch that made it easy to see exactly where I was going, and when the road turned up. Before I knew it I was climbing and feeling surprisingly good. Every little while, I'd pass Grandpa, give him the thumbs up and keep climbing. The canyons made for some interesting scenery and helped pass the time. After awhile Grandpa asked how I was feeling, and I was able to respond, "Feeling good, I think I'll keep going."

After 35 miles, I came to the intersection where I would meet up with the family I was staying with that night. That is where I met the mom, Julie, and her four kids, Steven, Abbey, Lindsey, and Katie. They were a military family and really reminded me of my family. The four little blonde kids were home schooled, had a lot of energy and wanted to play when we got back to their house, so we did, while we ate fresh cantaloupe.

Later their dad, Steven Sr., came home and we ate spaghetti and talked about Colorado. They told me stories about how they have a friend there who built a rock wall in his staircase! That gave me some ideas for my home decorating future. Relaxing that night was nice and it felt a lot like being at home. Little Steven would come out of his room with a toy he wanted to show me and we'd play with it for about 5 minutes, he'd get tired of it and then bring out another; and then he brought out the Nintendo Wii. He wanted to play the Yoga game on Wii Fit so we all took turns sitting on the mat and had a competition of who could sit still for the longest. I lost and Steven won by a landslide. But in my defense, my legs wouldn't fold all the way to fit on the mat.

As we were playing, Steven their dad asked me if I listened to music while I ran. I informed him that I had an iPod shuffle that I brought along on the trip but it died, for the 8th and last time two days before I started. He told me that he bought all these cheap little MP3 players because he listens to them when he works out but they die pretty quickly due to submersion in sweat. They told me that the direction I was heading was going straight into the desert and there was over 100 miles of nothing. There were no gas stations, no buildings, no fire hydrants, not even a 7-11 and I was probably going to need something to take my mind off the monotony; so he gave me one of those little MP3 players. Their taste in music was slightly different than mine, but they had Guns and Roses, Whitesnake, and Pink Floyd on their computer. He loaded it onto the computer and even gave me extra batteries! That MP3 player lasted me not only through the desert and out of California but all the way to Tybee Island, Georgia.

CHAPTER 16

The next morning they drove me a couple miles to where I had left off the day before and we unloaded my stroller and gear. They signed my banner while I assembled my rig and I overheard Steven ask his mom, "Mom, is Patrick staying with us tonight too?"

"No, Steven, not tonight."

"Well then, when?"

"I'm not sure, but someday."

Then Steven gave me a little license plate with his name on it. It was a little plastic Nevada plate so I tied it to the back of my stroller where I could see it all the time; and there it stayed.

I liked this family. They were good people, and I enjoyed their company. When I heard Steven ask his mom when I was coming back it struck a chord in me. Even though I had been on the road less than a week, the lack of familiarity played strange games with my emotions. I felt attached to every family I came in contact with whether I had a lot in common with them, or nothing at all.

I had an interview with the newspaper of the Marine Corps Base 29 Palms that I was to meet with at an intersection 14 miles away. That would be roughly my halfway point for the day and it would be a good time to stop to take a break. There happened to be a McDonalds there and since I got there early I decided to go in and refill my bottles and sit on the bench there. When I came out, the kids and Julie were there to visit. Apparently, during their school day the kids kept asking where I was and so Julie decided since they weren't staying focused, they would embark on a field trip.

The time came for the interview and a young private came out to do the interview. He was incredibly polite and was a great interviewer. Bill, whose house I would stay that night, and I worked out a time to be picked up and I was on my way.

After about 10 blocks, I was out in the desert. Every so often there would be a small house and some of them had huge fences with barbed wire around them and big guard dogs who didn't like me. I didn't know what they were doing in the houses with the fences. Whatever it was, they didn't want visitors.

Being in the desert was like nothing I had ever experienced. The view stretched on for miles and miles. Tiny shrubs and even tumbleweeds were not uncommon but even the things that were technically plants looked dead and barren. Hills were more like giant rock piles that some giants had produced just for fun. It was very flat but the terrain seemed to roll on and on until a pile of rocks interrupted the flow of flatness. Just north of where the road was, there was pile of rocks that resembled a mountain ridge. It wasn't very high, maybe a couple hundred feet, but it just seemed to go on forever in both directions. I thought maybe if I could get up to the top of the ridge and if I didn't have to push the stroller, it might be more interesting to run up there rather than the treadmill-like run on a black ribbon through the sandy landscape. It was slow moving, but it was moving.

I heard the loud engine of a Mustang coming up behind me signaling that my ride was here. Cruising through the desert in a Mustang is not a bad way to travel and caused me to ask myself why I was running as opposed to riding in a fast car.

Bill had come to pick me up and drive me to his house in his beast of a car. He knew a lot about the desert and adventure races. We got talking about them and he and his son hike a lot in the nearby mountains. When I got to their house I met Bill's three kids and his wife Vicki. Everyone was very welcoming. They must have heard that I ate a lot because they made a massive amount of food. Chicken and broccoli was on the menu that night and was absolutely delicious. It really hit the spot. It was very relaxing being with the family, unfortunately, being out in the dry heat all day I was exhausted very early. I figured I should go to sleep early.

That night I kept waking up for no reason and had trouble getting back to sleep. This was about the time I stopped sleeping regularly. I figured I only got about four hours of sleep that night, but woke up the next morning not feeling tired. It was frustrating but in the first few weeks, I would not sleep well for a couple nights and then crash hard and sleep in a mini-coma for a long time. As time went on, the mini-coma crashes occurred fewer and fewer times until I was only sleeping 3-5 hours per night every night with no crash. It was very strange and yet was a pattern of sleeplessness I'd experience for the remainder of the trip.

Before I left the next morning I said goodbye to everyone who was awake. Bill gave me a giant bottle of sun screen. I felt it strange, because I didn't need it at all that day. It was so chilly and windy I needed a long sleeved shirt and opted for the SmartWool base layer. I started off down the road and soon ran out of things to look at. I felt good in the morning but before long, my Achilles tendon started to ache. It drove me crazy but was forcing me to walk a lot of the time. This was the day that my grandpa would meet up with me in his RV and stay with me; two guys out on the road, roughing it . . . with an RV. It would be an adventure I was looking forward to because my grandpa has always lived on the West Coast and I've always lived on the East Coast. I would see him from time to time, but for the most part the visits never lasted more than a week.

I started the run that morning with the stroller and when my grandpa caught up to me, I would throw the stroller on the bike rack he had on the front of his RV and I wouldn't have to push it again for a month; not until the first town in Texas: Plains. My Achilles kept hurting and the more I ran, the more it hurt. So I started walking. After about 10 minutes of walking, my grandpa pulled up and I put the stroller on the RV.

I was happy to see my grandpa. He is about 5' 8" medium built, with glasses and almost no hair. He is my mom's dad which means I'll have the same haircut soon enough. He was raised in Philadelphia and became an engineer, and helicopter pilot in the Army. Athletic by nature, he played soccer and baseball very well and for most of his life. He was also invited to try out for the Phillies when he was fresh out of high school. He and my grandma moved a lot with their three kids because of the Army. The eldest is my mom, Susie. My uncle Bob is the marathoner and husband to Vickie the Great. And Rich is the youngest brother whom you will meet in Alabama.

I was glad to get rid of the stroller, and I was hoping that it would help to solve my Achilles problem. Unfortunately, it didn't. That day was long and frustrating. After 30 miles I called it a day, still in pain from the Achilles. My grandpa was a bit worried because when he used to play soccer he tore his Achilles and knew that it could be a serious issue.

Due to being out in the desert, there was no cell phone coverage and so there was no way Katie could cheer me up tonight. A shower was also a no go due to the nature of where we were. It was funny how much a shower renews and refreshes you after a long day of running. It was okay because since it was so chilly that day, I didn't sweat much.

That evening we watched the sun set. It was incredible. Bill had said, "The desert was the best place in the world for sun rises and sun sets." He wasn't kidding.

My grandpa and I decided that since I wasn't shaving, he wasn't shaving. I had a three day head start on him, but he had a 50 year head start on beard growing capabilities.

CHAPTER 17

When I started running the next day it took 22 miles to get warmed up and for my Achilles to stop hurting. After it stopped though, I felt great.

I also was stopped by the police. Grandpa was leapfrogging about every 3-5 miles and in between one of the stops I was running along and a cop whizzed past me going the same direction. After about ten seconds I see the break lights go on and thought, "Oh great, that's all I need." They turned around and drove toward me. They slowed down to about 30 yards from me and turn on the loudspeaker.

"Are you alright?" They said very slowly like they weren't expecting me to be coherent.

I just gave a thumbs up.

"We just wanted to make sure your girlfriend didn't kick you out of the car."

These guys were alright by me.

They turned around and headed up the road the same direction I was going in. Then I saw their lights go on and pull in behind the RV that was still about 4 miles away (I could see about 50 miles in every direction where I was). I tried to run a little faster to get there to back up the wacky story the police would hear when Grandpa told them of my quest.

By the time I reached the RV they were gone but Grandpa had given them the business cards that told people what I was doing. He said they were cool and were just making sure he was okay too. They were a couple of good guys.

After 30 some miles we called it a day and Grandpa looked up in his RV book that a campground wasn't too far from where we were (in driving terms). We decided we would stay there.

While driving there we saw a couple of guys running in blue shirts. I knew I had been running in the desert for a couple days now but I was pretty sure I wasn't imagining them. We pulled up ahead and a whole bunch of "blue shirts" and a van were parked up ahead. We stopped to talk to them.

"Hi, we saw two guys in the same shirts running a ways back. What are you doing out here?"

"The taller guy, Mike, is part of the *Cures Rock! Team* and is running to Phoenix for cancer research," a woman in a matching blue shirt answered sounding a bit rehearsed.

The main runner, Mike, was running 30 miles a day along pretty much the same route except from San Diego to Phoenix for the Rock and Roll Phoenix Marathon to raise money for Cancer. The only difference was that he had started one day before I did. After Mike showed up they told me they had seen me on the news and referred to me as "stroller-guy," except I wasn't running with my stroller at the moment.

I was a little jealous of his entourage. He had a van going with him the entire way, a coach with him, a pacer with him some of the time and lots and lots of *the ladies* to cheer him on. Not too shabby, Mike. Since then, he has broken the Guinness Book Record for "Most miles run in a week."

Also thrown into the mix were two little girls, Summer and Autumn. They were the two Girl Scouts that had run with me out of the mall on the first day, both keeping up with me for a lot longer than I expected. The girls and their mom had driven over an hour from their house on a lake to come visit me in the desert. I could not thank them enough. To see a couple of familiar faces was nice. This outward kindness of almost complete strangers toward me would come to be a very large part of the trip that I appreciate more and more every time I think about it.

By this time in the trip, my dad had taken on the second full time job of managing everything for me. He seemed to know how to do everything from contacting newspapers, radio, and TV stations to contacting the towns' chamber of commerce and managing the inflow of money in a way that wouldn't get us in trouble with the IRS later. He was at it non-stop, and I'm not sure he slept for 4 months.

An RV park is something I think everyone needs to experience at least once in their lifetime. It isn't bad by any means, just something different. Some people live there full time, some are just passing through. Most are over the age of 65 and all are at least 50. There are dogs being walked, and golf carts driven. At any given time, at least half are being cooked in, and the thing to do is talk to people on your way to and from the shower house about how big your rig is and where you're from. Like I said, it's interesting place; needs to be experienced.

I was able to reach Katie that night, which was good. While I was walking around outside talking to her I heard an owl catch a rabbit or a hare and kill it. It was just something else I hadn't experienced.

CHAPTER 18

We drove back to where I left off the day before and I started running. It was nice to have seen everything that I would be seeing during the day so I knew what was coming up and what I was to look for when I was getting close to the end. While in the desert, though, there is only so much you can look for as far as landmarks go.

When I was getting nearer to the little general store where I met up with the *Cures Rock! Team* the previous day, a car stopped and it was Mike's coach, Bill from the Leukemia and Lymphoma Society. He stopped to give me some Gatorade and encouragement. He also told me I was limping quite a bit. Though my Achilles was still store, I was glad he told me so I could make a conscious effort not to. It seems whenever I limp, I tend to mess up whatever side I'm overcompensating with.

His encouragement and Gatorade worked because even though I was still about 10 miles from the Arizona border I picked it up and felt better. I guess there weren't many other roads nearby that crossed the Arizona border because there was a huge increase in large trucks along this stretch of road and I noticed it more because the shoulder narrowed significantly.

At the end of 30 miles I crossed the Colorado River into Arizona. One state down and I hadn't broken anything yet.

January 11th, was my 10th day. It was my first off day and I wasn't a fan of being so unproductive. Grandpa and I drove just north of where we were to Lake Havasu City, AZ and saw the original London Bridge. They had brought it over piece by piece and reassembled it as a tourist attraction.

The area was nice, and there was a killer Chinese Buffet that we decided we needed to put out of business by eating more than our body weight in cheap Chinese food. Finding buffets would soon become a goal when it came to reaching my caloric needs for the day.

My overall feeling on the day off was negative because I felt tired and unmotivated to do much of anything all day; not to mention it was another day I was out on the road without accomplishing any miles that day. My dad assured me that my body needed a break and as much as I hated it, it was still probably a good thing.

CHAPTER 19

When I started running it was very cold and I felt sluggish and unmotivated. It could've been the prior off day, the cold weather, the harsh wind, or the Chinese food I ate at noon the previous day. Possibly a combination of all of the above, but that didn't help my situation much right then.

The Arizona scenery had changed. Instead of seeing nothing but sand, the occasional shrub, and piles of rocks, now I saw more shrubs that looked brittle and half dead along with the sand and piles of giant rocks.

When I reached the town of Bouse, Arizona, my supposed stopping point, I ate a couple of peanut butter and jellies and decided to keep going because there was no point in stopping at 1 pm. What were we going to do for the rest of the day?

I added another 10 and called it a day.

In many of the towns in Arizona they put the first letter of the town in rock on one of the hills around the town. Since there are no large trees, it's very easy to see the towns' initial up there.

Here's another interesting tid-bit of information for you: They put advertisements on the side of tractor trailers and park the trailer right there on the side of the road. Thanks to this innovative way of advertising, I was able to get a good phone number for someone who will clean my septic tank if I ever own a house with a septic tank in Bouse, Arizona.

CHAPTER 20

The next few days were slightly uneventful, except I did pass a sign that said, "Your now passed all Hope," and it was spelled exactly like that, grammatical errors and all. It referred to an intersection that the map called a "town." I kept logging the miles, and Grandpa was with me the whole time. Most of the towns we went through had populations in the triple digits. A lot of them were nothing more than an intersection in the road with an old gas station that may or may not have still been in business.

I was still taking things one day at a time. It seemed to be working to keep me optimistic. Every once in a while, though, I would forget to *not* think about the mileage and a huge "2400 miles" would pop into my head. Sometimes I would think about the finish, and what it would feel like to run into the Atlantic Ocean. I thought about who might be there and what Tybee Island looked like.

My sleeping habits were still very strange, but I didn't seem to be breaking down, so I didn't think too much of them. I would lay awake at night and just look out the window to see whatever was new around us. Or I would think, as if I didn't have enough time to do that already. I spent a lot of time thinking over the course of the trip, but unfortunately, never came up with any answers to the big world problems. I guess I would have to keep running to see what else came to mind.

Chapter 21

The route I was still on was following pretty closely to I-10 and it was working well for the most part. Unfortunately, sometimes we ran out of paved road. I was a fan of this, but Grandpa and the RV weren't. I could only imagine seeing the inside of it while it's barreling down the gravel and dirt road; everything on the inside swinging open, food and supplies flying, and nothing staying in its place. It was also very dusty, and that part wasn't fun.

Trying to breathe when it would get hot and dusty seemed like more of a chore than something my body did on instinct. I just tried to hold my breath for a couple seconds every time a big car or truck rolled past. Luckily, there weren't many of those because the roads we were on were more like access roads than main roads.

As we approached Phoenix, I noticed that commercial buildings were not any more common. I was expecting commerce to start popping up little by little but when I got to my stopping point the day before I'd end in Phoenix; there still wasn't a whole lot around.

When we got to the end of the day, we decided to drive ahead and see Phoenix. I would be running into downtown the next day, but we wanted to see the city today. Another reason to go was that the Rock N Roll Phoenix Marathon was having their race expo over the next few days. We figured it would be a good opportunity to go and pass out business cards and get some publicity to hopefully raise some money.

We went into the convention center where the expo was being held. It was the standard race expo; vendors with stands, packet pick-up for the racers, race memorabilia for sale, and someone talking over the volumes of people piling in and out of the huge open space. I looked at the schedule of people who were giving little talks or seminars and I recognized one of the names. It was Dean Karnazes, author of *Ultramarathon Man*. I made my way over to the stage where various people would speak that day and he was speaking as I walked up. He was giving a little informational talk on how to recover quickly from running a marathon. I couldn't help but listen intently, because I too wanted to be able to recover quicker from running a marathon or more. Unfortunately for me, the secret he was giving away was one I was currently living by: run the next day, no matter what.

I waited for him to finish his speech and got in line for "autographs." The line was long, but I wanted to tell him who I was so that I could maybe get a mention on his blog for the Runner's World Magazine web site. I thought that would surely generate a hit or two to my website and possibly a couple bones toward the pile of cash we were raising for the Arthritis Foundation.

When it was my turn to talk to him, I walked up in my yellow "Patrick's Coast to Coast Run" shirt and said,

"Hi, my name is Patrick McGlade and I'm running across the country for Juvenile Arthritis."

He replied, "Yea, I heard about you, you're pushing the baby jogger right?"

I came clean about my Grandpa helping me through the barren parts of the country and we only spoke for a minute or two about ultra running and the likes because the line was still long behind me. My dad had just finished his book on the plane ride out to California and was very impressed, so I got him an autograph and mailed it home the next day.

Grandpa and I looked around the expo for the *Cures Rock! Team* but couldn't find them. As we were looking around I started talking to this guy that worked for Youth Juice. It's a type of juice that helps your body replace what it lost during a long run quicker. It has lots of antioxidants and all that good stuff to help you stay healthy. After we talked for awhile, he said that if I wrote about Youth Juice on my blog that night, then I could have a bottle for free to try.

Since that was a deal I couldn't refuse, I took the bottle and wrote about it that night. It ended up tasting delicious and after looking at the ingredients just realized that it was all berries, fruit and herbs; standard herbs; not the "special" herbs.

71

After giving out a stack of business cards at the expo, we decided to call it a day and head back to the area I ended the day in. That night we stayed in a hotel that the local Arthritis Foundation of Arizona had gotten for us. We would have loved to meet them but with their events that were coming up, they were very understandably busy.

Sleeping in a real bed was incredibly comfortable and I slept well that night.

Chapter 22

I was excited the next day to run into the downtown area of Phoenix. The exact spot I was finishing was right in the middle of downtown and right next to the convention center the expo was held in. As I ran that day the sights around me slowly started to get more populated and more concrete started popping up. I ran past construction and saw it as a sign that the city was growing.

I could see downtown's tall office buildings in the distance as I entered the west side of Phoenix. It was almost like I crossed a country's border. Immediately all the signs were in Spanish and the only language I heard around me was Spanish. While I was standing at a stoplight waiting to cross, a guy yelled out his car window, "Hey man! Your shorts are too short!" I assumed he hadn't seen many runners around this part of the city and just ignored it. At the next stop light a homeless guy was sitting on the corner and asked me who I was running from. I told him,

"The west coast."

"You mean like, the Atlantic Ocean?!"

"No, the Pacific Ocean. I'm running TO the Atlantic Ocean."

"Oh crap, man, don't you get hungry? I'm hungry and I'm just sitting here."

"You want a couple granola bars?"

"What's a granola bar?"

I pulled two out of my pack and gave it to him. "Just try it, you'll like it."

"Alright, I'm trusting you, now."

"Don't worry, it's good, and you won't be hungry for awhile. I'll see you later; I've got to keep going."

As I started to run across the street away from his corner he shouted,

"Thanks dude! And hey! Tell me what Minnesota looks like!"

I called over my shoulder, "Will do!" and was on my way.

Entering the actual city was exciting for me. It was the first major city I hit since being in Huntington Beach. It reminded me of running around Richmond, Virginia, where I went to school and did most of my training. The city didn't look all that different and the people didn't look much different.

That night, I stayed at the St. Francis Retreat House. It is a retreat house that is set up more like a retreat village and is nestled into the side of a very rocky hill. The Catholic Church is in the front of the village and doubles as the front wall. Then along the side of the church, is the main office, then the dining hall is next to that on the right. Behind all of this, are the rooms, and the gardens. Beautiful gardens, all of it desert themed, which was probably a result of being in a desert climate. It made the walk from the office to the rooms a very pleasurable venture.

My contact there was a man by the name of Charlie. I spoke with him several times in emails and on the phone coordinating my visit, but I only got to speak with him for a few minutes when I was there.

The retreat is mainly run by the Franciscan priests and every person I met there was very kind. I spent the evening in the gardens reading and enjoying the cool evening air.

The next morning, Grandpa and I attended the mass there and then returned to the city for my run that day. The issue we had to get around was that it was a lot of other people's running day as well. It was Sunday, and the Rock and Roll Phoenix Marathon was going on, right where I needed to go.

CHAPTER 23

On the drive there, we studied the race course and my course and tried to figure out the best way to get around thousands of people. We also had to figure out how to get the RV around all the people without me running out of water.

As we looked at the map of where I would go, and the courses of where the marathon and half marathon would go, it suddenly dawned on us, if you can't beat them, join them. I would run to the course and simply join in the half marathon race at around their 8 mile mark, finish the race with all of those people, make my way out of the finish line area, continue my run on my own and meet up with Grandpa just off the highway that goes around the city: the route that he would take. It seemed like there was a lot of room for error, but we didn't really have much of a choice so we each went our separate ways with the same ending point in mind.

The run down to the race course was only a couple of miles, but it was kind of awkward. There were a lot of people who were spectators for the race, and I got all sorts of funny looks from people walking around. I think it was because there was a very obvious running event just ahead of me, but I was clearly not part of it.

Before I knew it I had reached the race course. There was a wall of spectators about 5 people deep right where I needed to get into the mix. I said "excuse me," but no one seemed to care, they just kept clapping and screaming for the runners. Big signs that said, "Run till you Die!" and "Run Forest Run!" bounced above the spectators. I guess they were pretty serious about this. I said, "Excuse me!" again louder, and one guy with a giant handlebar moustache turned around and said, "What makes you think you're going to see your runner any better from where you are?"

I decide to pick a different spot to penetrate the wall of people. When I found a weak spot in the wall, I squirmed through the few people that were there and stood in front for a second or two acting like I was waiting for my runner to come along. I saw some guy with a shirt that said, "TOM" on it. I acted like he was my runner and yelled, "Hey Hey! Way to go Tom!!" and ran up to him acting like I knew the guy. He gave me a funny look like, "Do I know you?" But by that point I was already in the race running with the rest of the competitors. I left Tom, but I don't think he was too upset about it.

There were a ton of people running where I joined in but it was a fun atmosphere. There were people lining the street and horns buzzing, Gu, the nutritional packet of deliciousness, being handed out (like I didn't have enough of that already) and water cups handed to me by volunteers in latex gloves every mile or so. I had it made! We all ran the course, following the sea of people in front of us blindly around turns and up hills. If the course had led us off a cliff, we wouldn't have known until we were already falling. As we approached the finish line people were losing their minds screaming for us as we were "almost there." I couldn't help but think, *No I'm not. I still have 6 more states left*. We all crossed the finish line and one guy turns to me in between huge gasps of breath and gives me a high-five saying, "Sweet man! I can't believe I just did that." I was happy for him. It was the sheer thrill of conquering a new distance. He went further than he ever had in his life, and he could not only breathe afterward, but he could walk, and talk about it. There was a look of bliss, and yet a calm proud kind of smile spread across his sweat-soaked face. He conquered something that, I think, he might have had doubts about before this very moment. As selfish as it sounds, I hoped that I could have that same feeling very soon.

Just as I was thinking this, someone came up to me and started to put a medal around my neck. I said, "No, Thank you." I was a race bandit, and I didn't even run the whole race, I didn't want to take the medal. Besides, I'd have to lug one more thing around in my jogger. Going through the finish line area provided me with many snacks. I had to take full advantage of the opportunity to get fed. I stuffed granola bars and bananas into my pack and made my way to areas less crowded.

I found the street I was supposed to be on and followed it east. It just so happened that the marathon was heading west on the same road and was in the last 5 miles. I was able to see a lot of people at the end of their race, and I even saw Pam Reed, elite ultra marathoner, winner of the Badwater Ultra marathon two years in a row, and the race director for the Tucson Marathon.

After a couple miles I met up with Grandpa and continued on my day's run. I had families to stay with the next two nights and it was in a slightly strange situation with the mileage because the houses where I was staying were both close to each other and were closer to where the end of the race was—behind me. I know that having the RV with us made it easier to get to a house that was further away, but at the same time, mentally, running further and further away from where you're staying makes it difficult to come up with a reason to keep going that day.

I finally got to the end of my day and we drove to where I was staying that night. Danelle, Dan, and their daughter, Ashley greeted me at the door, along with their dog, Winny. He was an incredibly energetic puppy and was the size of a full sized dog. He just wanted some love, and I was just the man for the job. He was also very curious of what was in my bag. I decided that he would be a great dog to run with, but his family was rather attached to him, and Grandpa didn't seem too fond of him. Ashley had Juvenile Arthritis herself, and unfortunately didn't have it under control. She had not yet found a medication that worked. And after telling me she had tried almost all of them, I was frustrated for her. I couldn't imagine how she felt about it. I was glad she told me about her battle with JRA but was disappointed for her that nothing had seemed to work yet.

For dinner that night we had the most heavenly concoction of Mexican glory I had ever tasted. She asked me if I had ever had enchiladas. I said "yes." She asked, "But have you ever had MY enchiladas? The real way?" I couldn't reply the same way.

It was settled. We were having enchiladas. "The real way."

Along with enchiladas she made homemade bread. I was ready to eat like a king. And her building up the reputation of her enchiladas didn't help to suppress my appetite. They were almost ready and she asked, "Would you like an egg on top?"

"An egg? Like a chicken egg? On enchiladas? Is that the way you eat it?"

"Sure is!"

"Alright then, I think I'll try an egg on top."

She then asked Grandpa, "Grandpa, you want an egg too?"

He looked at me and hesitated, "I think I have to try this, I'm not sure when I'll get another chance."

When we sat down and I looked at the plate in front of me, I could see ground beef, beans, lettuce, salsa and a big ol' fried egg plopped right on top of it all. I was a bit skeptical, but then again, there isn't much I don't like in terms of food, and by "not much" I really mean there's nothing I don't like.

I took one bite and the flavors mixed in with my taste buds. Let me begin to try to explain how awesome this thing tasted. Actually, I can't. It was that good. This giant pile of food, which only a few minutes earlier had me questioning the nature of the people I was staying with that night, was now gone and I was wondering what made that heavenly blend of unlikely foods the Mona Lisa of foods I had encountered in my lifetime up to this point at age 21. I sat there wondering if I had consumed some sort of food deity that the ancient Mexican people bowed down to. I wanted to know so that I too, could bow before thine heavenly plate of the divine enchiladas with egg on top.

The next day, the enchiladas fueled me well and made me feel like a million bucks. There was one slight problem for the day: I ran out of road. Grandpa and I looked at the map and saw that the road continued to go straight, yet where we were standing, the road clearly ended. Had I been a wuss, I might not have taken the opportunity to get my feet a bit dirty and would've turned around and stuck to the pavement. Nope, not today, I would keep to my trail roots and bushwhack my way to the other side, where I was supposed to go. Grandpa turned around and stuck to the roads. As awesome as it would've been to see an RV catch air off the dirt mounds I was about to cross, that adventure would be best saved for another day and another RV. Besides, if we wrecked the RV, Grandpa might have been stuck running across the country with me, and I only had one baby jogger.

Sure enough, the road connected on the other side, and I met up with Grandpa and continued the run no problem. As I would pass the RV every so often, most times Grandpa would be outside with some sort of food or to ask me how I was doing. And at the end of the day, he'd stand outside and clap for me like I had finished a race. When I saw the RV for the last time in the distance, signaling my finishing point for the day, I noticed I didn't see the now scruffy man outside. I got closer and still, just the RV. I figured it was a bit too chilly for the thin-blooded southern Californian and he must have just been keeping warm inside.

When I opened the door I found what had been keeping him from giving me my usual half-joking round of applause for finishing another day. *Maury*. He had found a TV station that was broadcasting *Maury* and they had just done the paternity test, and he needed to know who the "baby daddy" was. *Maury* read the words to seal the fate: "You are NOT the father." My grandpa started laughing hard. Shaking his finger at the TV he said, "I knew it! I knew it!" I didn't know of my grandpa's guilty pleasure, but now that I knew, there would be many jokes to come.

Kelly and her son Austin lived relatively close to where I stayed the previous night. Kelly was a college friend of Catherine's, who I met back in California on the 2nd day. Catherine had called Kelly and asked if I could stay with her and Austin and she immediately welcomed me.

When Kelly invited me, she put out a message to her Facebook friends, and that's where Danelle came in the previous night. They were friends and it just so happened, that Danelle's daughter, Ashley had arthritis, and so she invited me in last night. It's funny how my places to stay were often linked together by different people.

They had a puppy as well and he was very well behaved, except for his love of chewing shoes; so I was warned to keep my shoes out of reach. Austin was in middle school and ran cross country and played baseball. They had a ping pong table and I was able to see if Grandpa was really as good as he said he was.

Turns out, he was. Nothing got by him.

Austin's dad came over for dinner and we had a very nice time.

CHAPTER 24

It was time for my second day off, and McKemy Middle School was the first school I visited to talk to kids about the run. Austin attended school there, so Kelly set it up where I would be able to hang out with the gym teachers and talk to every class that came in. Each class had about 30-50 kids in it, and Austin was in the first class, so it was good to see a semi-familiar face. I spoke to 6 different periods and every time got a little easier than the last. I expected the kids to be sort of rowdy and not very receptive. I couldn't have been more wrong. Not only were they well behaved, but they asked some great questions. It's great to see how kids' brains work, because I realized it's not too far off how mine works. Among my favorite questions were,

"What's your favorite kind of jelly for pb&j's?"

"Do you sleep?"

"Where do you go to the bathroom?"

"When you push the baby jogger, whose baby will you put in there?"

Usually, my little segment of the class didn't last the whole period, but there wasn't enough time to start an activity so the coaches put on the radio and the kids played basketball. During one of the periods, the radio came on and it was "Single Ladies" by Beyonce. This 7th grade boy just started doing the dance that Beyonce does in the song. It was hilarious, so I took a video and stuck it on the blog.

During the lunch break, I got to know the coaches a little better. Coach Benson used to do gymnastics and was really good. We got talking and he, too, was a valet. He told me about this one time he was at work and he sprinted to a car. When he reached the car, it was really nice and when he returned the car, the owner looked at him and said, "Man, I've never seen a white boy run like you." Turns out, the owner of the car was Jesse Owens.

CHAPTER 25

Weather can be a funny thing, and so can mountains. Mountains can have their own weather patterns, completely separate from the flatlands though the two may only be a few miles apart.

The past couple days we had been watching a series of storm systems go through the area called Show Low, Arizona; right where I was headed. The elevation was around 8,000 ft up there and I would be turning north a couple miles from where my run ended today in Globe—unless the snow got too bad. As Grandpa and I followed the radar of the storms we saw them slam the area repeatedly, we worried that the route through Show Low would be impassable and we would have to reroute. The biggest issue we had was that the alternate route was impossible to run without running on I-10 for 50 some miles, with random secondary and service roads in between for a few miles here and there.

My dad wrote to the police department up in Show Low to try to get an idea of what the conditions were from someone experiencing them as they were happening. We received updates every morning on how much snow they actually got the night before and how much had melted the previous day. At one point it was snowing 2 or 3 feet every night for 3 days.

I wasn't worried about running in it, but the concern was the RV and the lack of 4 wheel drive, and chains.

The conditions were harsher than the news made it out to be and we were incredibly fortunate to get a pair of eyes on the ground to help us make our decision when the time came. The information we received was invaluable and I owe a great deal of my safety in this portion of the run to the Show Low Police Department. We would have to make a decision in the next day or so, but I had to get to Globe—my fork in the road—first.

CHAPTER 26

I started on my run the day I'd end in Globe. I started uphill and remained that way for quite awhile. Then I went downhill for a long time. Then up, then down. And I repeated this for most of the morning. What I didn't realize was that while I was going down, I wasn't going down as much as I was going up. The scenery was stunning each time I came to a little peak and the whole way down was incredibly enjoyable.

After a little while, we went through the little town of Miami nestled in between two mountains. I entered the town, and 5 minutes later I was exiting the town.

I could see that the road in front of me curved up; straight up. I decided to power hike most of this section to save my energy for later. The road curved, and I remained leaning forward hiking up the road. There were semi-trucks pulled over, some with smoking engines from trying to climb the steep grade. Then I noticed that a lot of the semi's that were passing me were not going too much faster than I was. I started running a little bit and realized that I could keep the same pace as a semi while climbing this mountain. I was racing semi-trucks to the top of the mountain. What's up ego boost?

After another hour of climbing, I caught up to where Grandpa had pulled over to wait for me. He pulled into the run-away ramp because there wasn't a shoulder to pull over on due to narrow, winding roads. The spot where he pulled off was right next to my first obstacle for the day—a tunnel.

Cars came screaming down the mountain and barreling through the tunnel at high speeds. The cars and trucks that were climbing the mountain were crawling through the dark tunnel. The combination of the two made Grandpa nervous for my safety and offered to drive me through the quarter mile hole in the mountain. Of course, I didn't want to be driven because then I would have run across the whole country except for this little spot. We came to the conclusion that because it looked like the tunnel flattened out, I would sprint through the tunnel and he would follow me through in the RV, thus, blocking one lane of the two lane traffic. I took a break and ate and drank so I'd have enough energy to get through the thing at the break-neck speed I was hoping for.

When we were both ready, I started. I put my head down, and stared at the ground as my legs churned and chugged as fast as they could. I didn't want to look up to see how much longer I had or see cars careening down the mountain at me. Besides, a very large part of me was scared that the "light at the end of this tunnel" was not going to be the kind of light I was hoping for. My breathing got heavier, and my arms pumped and I couldn't help but think, "This is not as flat as it looked." I had been going up for so long, my view of *flat* was skewed and I was sprinting up a steep incline. My head remained down. I stared at the white line passing under my feet as though this was my safety rope—the inanimate object that would carry me to safety. If the line was ever interrupted from the paint fading with time I felt as if my safety rope had frayed and I ran just a little faster. My heart felt like it was the raw knuckles of a boxer trying to fight his way out of my ribcage. Constantly pounding faster and stronger with every step, I was unsure how much faster my heart could possibly pump. I finally felt myself break back into daylight and jumped onto the side of the road so that Grandpa could pass me and the rest of traffic could get by.

Completely out of breath I walked toward the RV and Grandpa, who was standing outside now.

"That was a pretty good run!"

I looked back at the tunnel I had just traversed; it looked a lot more like a hill from up here. I could see the mountain above the tunnel. I pictured the designers coming to this mountain, scratching their heads and saying, "Nope, can't go over this one, might as well blast through it." And that's just what I did.

The rest of the day was in the foothills and mountains. I had an absolute blast climbing and descending all day. It should have been the tough in terms of elevation gain and loss, but it turned out to be the easiest because it was so interesting. The rock faces on each side looked like something from a painting of the "wild west." Then, ten minutes later, the scenery was completely different with a snow-capped giant off in the distance, with green grasses and trees growing everywhere.

The run ended in Globe, AZ. It was a 35 mile day and it felt good to finish, I also looked forward to more mountains coming in the next couple days.

That day, January 20th, also happened to be Grandpa's birthday! We found an RV campsite right next to a casino, so I took him into the casino for an all-you-can-eat feast.

The weather was also very nice, sunny, and cool.

Grandpa couldn't take the itchiness associated with the first couple days of beard growing, so he shaved that day as well. I was disappointed the tough old man wasn't quite up to challenge of growing a beard.

CHAPTER 27

We woke up that night at about 1 or 2 am and were absolutely freezing. We got up and turned on a little space heater that Grandpa had brought with us. I would have never thought to bring it, but he came prepared.

When we woke up the next morning it was raining a very cold rain. I decided to run anyway after a bit of a delay in the morning to wait to see if temperatures would rise above 33 degrees.

I started off in my full rain suit. After a little while, I made the turn to go north toward Show Low. There were signs that said, "Caution: Heavy snow up ahead. Chains REQUIRED."

I'm not sure why I kept running up those hills. We still weren't sure if we were going to go through Show Low or re-route, but I decided I didn't want to get too far behind just in case we did go north.

After a painstakingly slow run in the cold and wet rain, up and down the foothills of the mountains I was heading toward, I stopped. There was no point in it, and therefore, no motivation. I only went 15 miles in 3 hours and was utterly exhausted. My muscles didn't ache; I was just drained of energy. It was like the cold rain washed away any energy I had and even took the energy I didn't have.

We stayed at the casino RV park again that night. After taking a hot shower and skipping and jumping my way across the parking lot to avoid stepping in the growing puddles I crawled back into the RV and bunkered down for the evening next to the space heater.

Buried in the down sleeping bag I stared up at the ceiling of the RV where I could feel the heat from the space heater gently grace the left side of my face, I had never been so thankful that Grandpa had come with me. This situation could have been potentially life threatening if I didn't have a dry place to sleep. I realized all of this now, and especially when I woke up the next morning. At some point during the night, the storm that was hitting Show Low again, swooped down and hit us in Globe dropping the temperatures even lower and dumping a couple inches of snow on us. It was the first time Globe had seen snow in 2 years. And the day I was there, so was the snow.

The minute I saw the snow, I knew today was going to be a forced day off. It was incredibly frustrating. I hardly got anywhere yesterday and I wouldn't be going anywhere today. I was supposed to be in the mountains today! I was supposed to be cruising up and careening down steep pitches without a care in the world. I knew it would be cold, and there would be snow on the sides of the road, but why did there have to be this storm? Instead of staring in awe at 8,000-10,000 ft beauties, I was stuck in a parking lot of a casino and there would be a strong possibility of not ever getting to run through Show Low at all.

Reading was how we spent most of the morning. Bunkered down in the RV with just the pages of a book to try to burn some of my growing amounts of energy, I tried to distract my growing frustration with the story of some deep-sea adventure/mystery/comedy/conspiracy book. Unfortunately, it didn't work and I finally succumbed to the decision I hadn't wanted to make. If we wanted to move anywhere in the next week, we would have to reroute to take a more southern route. True: it wouldn't be as pretty of a run, the altitude was lower, the trees were smaller or non-existent, I would have to run on the highway and could potentially get thrown off the highway by the police, and the route was a bit longer. But at least I would be getting somewhere. So it was decided. In the morning, we would head south, toward Safford, AZ, and much of the route would be made up as we went using only the maps we had and the "Maps" app my iPhone had on it. It was some consolation to know that tomorrow I would be moving ahead. In reality, I just didn't want to stay at the casino another night. I was tired of being in the same place.

CHAPTER 28

The next morning was sunny and bright. The air was incredibly crisp and my breath could be seen whether I breathed out of my mouth or nose. Humidity was very low and so was the temperature. The new snow, though only a couple of inches, looked funny hanging off of palm trees and reflected the sun to the point it was almost blinding. The land that was once mostly brown with a slight bit of green thrown into the mix was now fresh and completely white. Yet, it was already starting to melt due to the sun being so strong.

I started running and was heading down a very straight road in the new direction of south. It felt good to have my legs again under me moving me forward. Every step felt like I was gaining something. I had lots of energy to burn, and it felt like I was fueled by the purest of fuels: laziness. My laziness from yesterday gave me a renewed sense of meaning to today's run.

I headed down the straight road at a slight incline; so slight you almost couldn't even tell it was there. About a quarter mile ahead, there was a pair of small guardrails that I assumed could only mean there was a small bridge under it. There was a little white pick-up truck humming along coming down the road toward me. As it hit the bridge, it swerved and before I could finish my current blink it headed toward the opposite side of the road's guardrail. It smashed into the guardrail with the rear right light hitting first and bounced back to the other side of the road and smashed the front left corner and stopped. I ran as fast as I could toward it and as I got closer I saw that the windshield had been cracked and would've been completely smashed had it not been shatter-proof. The car door opened slowly and a man stumbled out all bloody. He was bleeding from his forehead and shoulder. Just then two other cars drove up and one person yelled that he was on the phone with police.

I asked the guy, "Are you okay?"

"Aw man! This sucks!"

I repeated myself, "But are you okay?"

"Yea man, I'm fine."

Within 5 minutes the police had gotten there, and it was okay to leave. The guy who crashed was okay, except for a small slice on his eyebrow. He just wasn't used to driving on icy roads, but then again, no one in the area was.

I made my way up the road as it wound around hills, and sloped up and down. In the distance I could see the mountains where I would've been had we not re-routed. They were completely white with new fallen snow. I ran next to them all day and they seemed to taunt me, and made me wish we hadn't changed the route. Before long, we were past where the storm had hit, and there was no longer any snow around.

Towards the end of the day, new mountains presented themselves, grew in the distance, and before long, I was right next to them; running with giants. The hills surrounded me, and I kept rolling over them. Soon, though, a new view presented itself—storms. I could see three distinct storm cells around me and it took a minute to decide which ones were heading toward me. I was relieved to learn that none of them were, but that didn't make them any less fun to look at. Though none of them drenched me directly, the weather was strange that day. At the start, the weather was sunny and cold at 34 degrees. Then it was warm. Then rainy. Then cold. Then sleet made a guest appearance. Then a little hail. Then it came back full circle to sunny and cool.

Other than the strange spectrum of weather, it was a bit of a strange day in other areas as well. I saw three dead dogs, and four dead skunks. Not cool. 14 people honked at me. I'm not sure if it was because they've never seen anyone running or if I had some leftover peanut butter and jelly smeared on my face. Regardless, it was weird and I didn't taste any PB&J when I checked.

I also saw 11 hypodermic needles in about a quarter mile.

After 35 miles, I ended the day in Bylas.

CHAPTER 29

Day 23 brought with it clear skies; very clear blue skies. I started the day and felt good and had the feeling that the old legs needed a quicker run today. I picked it up a little bit and hit cruise control. I passed three hitch-hikers, "Who you running from man?"

I told them what I was doing but they didn't seem to believe me. The two guys and the girl were hitch-hiking their way to work, but it didn't look too promising for them. They had walked for the last 5 or so miles and only had another hour to finish the last 10 miles. I walked with them for a minute. Then I gave them some Gu Chomps because that's all I had with me and they said they were hungry. But then I said my goodbyes and resumed my run. About 40 minutes later they waved to me from the back of a pickup truck bed.

Next came the dogs.

I was running at a decent clip and three dogs started barking at me from their yard. Luckily, they were surrounded by barbed wire. They were going nuts and were running in circles around their yard; then they all changed directions and started toward the fence and jumped right through a hole in the barbed wire.

I slowed down a bit to hopefully show them that I wasn't threatening but I was getting a little nervous. Plus, I didn't want to book it because I wanted to keep an eye on these monsters. There weren't any cars around and these dogs were losing their minds. They got within about 15 feet of me and stopped to make a fan formation between me and their house.

One was snarling and moving slowly closer staying low in a semi-army crawl looking dangerously like he was ready to pounce. I backed away a little quicker.

90

The other two kept barking and were jumping around—still mad. When they were 4 feet away I just sort of stood in an uncomfortably strong position hoping they would be scared if I tried to act big and tough. For whatever reason, it seemed to work. I must be some sort of dog whisperer or something because the other two dogs calmed down a bit and the one stopped moving toward me.

Then, I simply backed away slowly and kept right on running. I have to admit, the acting tough thing was uncomfortable, and I don't expect it to ever work again, but I was glad it worked that day.

For the rest of the day I kept a decent pace and felt strong. Then, for whatever reason, my right thigh seized up and I got a monster cramp that forced me to walk. It was the weirdest thing but I figured something was out of balance so I drank some more water, ate a Gu, as well as an electrolyte tablet and kept running. It worked itself out and I was able to finish the 33.9 day in 4:54. For those days, that was a decent time for me. Normally I only timed the day so I had a record of when I should eat and things like that, but that day, I used it to race time.

That day was a complete shift in thinking for me. There was no logical reason why I should run any faster that day. I just woke up that day feeling competitive with myself.

The day ended right at the foot of a great looking mountain that looked like it needed to be climbed, but I resisted.

Chapter 30

There is a woman named Eva who is a part of the Virginia Happy Trail Runners Club, the same running club I am in. She had heard about the run and was going to California for a work conference. Eva wanted to come out to where I was and run a whole day with me. I didn't know her beforehand but she offered to come out, and I wasn't about to turn down the company. We made plans to meet up the next day.

Eva had driven 9 hours from California to run with me. I didn't know anything about her when we started running, except she was from Eastern Europe. I got that from her accent while talking about plans on the phone. When I met her at the gas station we had planned on, I met a vertically challenged woman with an equally small frame; short light brown hair cut in a semi-bowl cut, fair skin and was wearing a backpack as big as she was. We talked her into leaving the backpack in the car and just using the CamelBak; though it took some effort. She always ran with a giant backpack stuffed with anything she might need in the course of 100 miles.

It was very cold when we started but the air was clean and clear. I didn't mind the cold, and still ran in shorts, anticipating getting warm relatively soon after we started. Eva ran in running tights and several shirts; which I didn't learn until she started shedding the extra layers later on in the day revealing that her small frame was even smaller than I had originally thought.

Her English was very good, and she had a very large vocabulary, especially in the world of the sciences. That is because that's what she is: a scientist. She is not just any scientist; she is the awesome kind that pokes and prods rat's brains while they perform various tasks in a maze and motivates them with cheese. True, it sounds like the standard "mad scientist" but she was far from standard.

She was telling me about her research and what she was trying to prove, and it wasn't that I wasn't listening, but I don't remember a bit about it because her research was so advanced it just went straight over my head. It went in one ear and out it other, much like when my mom used to tell me to clean my room. Hearing stories from her childhood from Czechoslovakia and listening to how differently we were raised, not in ideals or morals, but in the culture aspect really taught me a lot in the 5 or so hours we ran together.

We ran next to the whole length of a small chain of mountains and then when it ran out, we kept running. We ran on a long stretch of road that was so straight and so long, I didn't want to take my eyes off the white line for awhile for fear that it wouldn't feel like I was getting any closer to the end of that road. Even after running a half of a mile, 5 minutes, I looked up and couldn't see any change in my point of view. We ran through an intersection of the road we were on and a road that would take me directly to the mountains I was supposed to be running in had the weather been better. It was hard not to turn north and trade the increasingly desolate landscape for one that was more densely populated with lush, green vegetation and large scenic mountains.

We continued along and every 4 miles or so Eva would eat her cheese sandwiches during our breaks at the RV. She helped motivate me, without saying anything, to not take many walking breaks, and I was even more motivated when we started talking about which races we each had dreams of running. For her, Hardrock 100 was at the top of her list; arguably the toughest 100 miler in terms of elevation change. For me—Badwater. We traded pros and cons of each race and realized that we each wanted to run every race we heard of; just to do it and see different courses in the process.

At the end of the day, she still looked fresh. She was a tough runner, and since then has done several ultras, including running an unmarked 100 miler, which she won, all while prodding her way to a sure scientific breakthrough in neuroscience. I was glad she ran with me that day and was disappointed she had to go. She kept great company but she wanted to see the Grand Canyon before she had to get back on her flight. I would've left me too in order to run in the Grand Canyon.

CHAPTER 31

Finishing the day with Eva also put me within running distance of New Mexico. Starting off the day, I was in pain, lots and lots of pain. Strange places, that I wasn't sure what to do to fix, hurt. The tendons in back of one knee pinched to an extreme biting feeling, the lower part of the opposite leg, the side of one hip; and the list went on and on.

There were several reasons I didn't do anything about it, or say anything to anyone. The first, and most important, was that it never hurt for more than one day. It seemed that the pain would be dull in the morning for whatever hurt. Then as the day went on and the blood started flowing more, the pain went away completely. Then towards the end of the day, it would come back very strong, borderline excruciating. By the time I ate my fill that night, got my couple hours of sleep, and woke up the next morning, it didn't hurt anymore. Injuries were starting, festering, going away, coming back with a vengeance, and healing completely within a 24 hour time period.

The other reason I didn't do anything about it was that every day it would be something different, and I don't like complaining too much. I think it's very annoying to hear myself complain. I can't imagine what I would sound like to someone else while I was whining. And the third reason is that I'm not a fan of painkillers, and if they are there and I don't want to take them, then I should just quit my whining, suck it up, and deal with it.

That day though, all I could do was try my best to forget I was running. I was trucking along staring at the white line, and doing my best to forget about moving and just try to think about something else. Unfortunately, the pains in my legs would not let me forget.

It was turning into a very low day as far as mentality goes. Getting hunted by more dogs didn't help me feel any less like a piece of lifeless meat plodding along the side of the road. They ran up, and I picked up a metal rod that looked like had come from a car and poked them away and it worked.

After what seemed like forever, I came to the sign that said, "Welcome to New Mexico." It was the most uneventful "finish of a state" I had.

I didn't care where I was or how much further I had to go. I just wanted to stop. My head remained low the entire day and I just kept moving.

All around me was desert.

The road was straight and slightly uphill for as far as I could see. As soon as I reached a point that revealed more road, it turned out to be more straight nothingness. I was demoralized. After a long day, I finished and was relieved. I was tired and didn't want to do anything but go to sleep even though it was early evening.

My grandpa drove to the closest town of Lordsburg, NM and tried to find a campground. We found a parking lot that was labeled as a campground. So we went in and got a space.

This parking lot was filled with people who had seen some misfortune in their day. There was an old bus that I assumed was transformed into some sort of motor home on the inside but I couldn't be too sure because the windows were just covered with sheets. They had an antenna springing from the top which was wrapped in aluminum foil. I heard a lot of yelling coming from inside and made me really uncomfortable. They had a dog tied to a stake just outside the door, which was running around in circles in the dust very quickly and never stopped barking as long as we were there. The windshield was cracked in several places and the back of the bus was held up with cinderblocks.

There were other RV's in the lot that had seen better days, and there was also a car that three guys slept in. It was a sad sight, and helped to put some of the things I had in perspective and made me thankful. Unfortunately, at that point, on that day, there was nothing that could improve my outlook on life.

We were told there was a shower around the back of the house in the back corner of the lot. I got all of my unmotivated energy together and gathered my showering supplies to make the trek across the parking lot in the cold wind to go wash away the bad day. When I reached the back of the building, it turned out there was no shower that I saw. I went back to the RV now shivering and informed Grandpa of our misfortune. I think he picked up on how terrible I was feeling and realized that I hadn't been sleeping well. While I entered the RV and got a snack, he left. After about 30 minutes he came back our little home and unplugged everything. I was confused but didn't ask any questions. I thought he was maybe going to fix something on the RV. Instead, he walked out the back door and climbed into the driver's seat and started the vehicle. He turned out of the decrepit parking lot and drove the couple blocks down the street to the motel. I was as happy as I could be right then and thanked him profusely. He said, "I think tonight you need a good night sleep. You weren't moving so well today."

When we arrived at the motel, I entered the bathroom and turned on the water. Thank God it was hot. From the looks of the motel, I wasn't so sure it would have hot water. I entered the shower that had lime build-up worse than I had seen in a long time, and black mold in all the corners. I didn't care at all. There wasn't much light to see because the light in the shower had burned out. Again, I didn't care. I put my face under the water and lost it. I think I cried harder than the water was coming out of the spout that was the same level as my head. This was hard, and I didn't like it. Today's run had been terrible. I felt dead and I didn't care about a thing. I didn't want to get out of the shower, I didn't want to go to bed, and I didn't want to take another step. My brain was fried, my legs were toast, and I couldn't come up with a single reason to stay out here.

The problem was I couldn't come up with a single reason to quit either. I couldn't imagine doing this for another couple months, but at the same time, I could measure my potential time left of being miserable. The kids that had arthritis on the other hand, couldn't say the same. They were waiting for an unknown amount of time for a cure, or to find a medication that would help to ease their pain. I realized this was my reason for staying out here. It was my reason for continuing the misery-fest and not calling it quits. It was my reason for staying so far from home and missing my family, friends and Katie like crazy. Though my finish line was still thousands of miles away, I had a finish line. The kids with arthritis don't. They are the reason I pulled myself together and didn't have Grandpa drop me off at the nearest airport the next day.

I was so thankful I got a shower and a bed that night. By getting us that room, Grandpa helped me more than he could possibly know, and more than I could tell him. He had saved the day.

Climbing into a real bed had never felt so good. The mattress was thin, and was incredibly springy. In hind sight, it was probably a grungy mattress with springs poking up everywhere and a dirty blanket, but for all I knew, it felt like multiple pillow-top mattresses with extra foam and an air pocket on top of clouds. I don't remember my head hitting the pillow; I think I was asleep before then. I just remember thinking as I got into bed, "Things can only get better from here."

CHAPTER 32

I woke up 11 hours later. It was the longest I had ever slept, and I felt much better. Starting off that day, I was much better mentally thanks to the shower and real bed I got to sleep in. It had revitalized me mentally, and physically. I was moving smoother, and feeling better. The scenery or lack thereof, was still bland but in the far, far distance I could see high mountains. It felt like something to look forward to, and that made me feel even stronger. I cruised through the straight roads section, and through Lordsburg.

I finally reached I-10 . . . again. This time, it was the end of my line. I had run out of secondary roads to take and I would have to run on the highway or next to it. I didn't think it would be legal to run on the highway so I opted to run in the dirt between the highway, and the barbed wire to keep people off the highway. I had to run 10 miles next this way and when I got to the end, I had to remove the huge, 1 to 2 inch thorns that had pierced the bottom of my shoes and poked into my feet.

The following day brought with it more highway sections. At first, I tried to run faster to spend less time on the actual road and hopefully that would result in less probability of getting stopped by the 5-0. It seemed to make sense in my head, but like any running related event, faster doesn't necessarily mean more efficient. I was able to stay on frontage roads but I did need to run on I-10 when the road ended. I knew there was a possibility of trouble so I ran fast. I had to cover 6 miles on the freeway and wanted to get it over with. I figured now would be a good time to work in some quicker speed work. But I guess my fear of someone kicking me off the highway and therefore skipping 6 miles of the whole country run had me running faster anyway.

It started raining out of nowhere and I was stuck trying to get to the RV before I was soaked to the bone; but it didn't work. By the time I reached my safe haven, I was so cold and wet that I was shivering semi-violently and couldn't feel my body. I had to open the door with two hands, and even then, I think Grandpa actually opened it from the inside. An hour and a half later, I was thawed out and put on warmer clothes and my rain clothes to battle the elements once again.

Soon after I left the RV I crossed the Continental Divide at 4,585 ft. For some reason, it felt like I had accomplished something once I crossed it, but I was still far away from the halfway point of the run, so the feeling of accomplishment was short lived.

As I was plodding along another section of I-10 in the rain and the head-on winds, I heard the sound of a siren and was somewhat relieved the police were going to tell me that I couldn't run here and make me get in their car because I was so tired from the thrashing I was getting from the weather. The cops pulled up behind me and a woman got out of the car. There was a guy cop as well, but he stayed in the car. I guess she drew the short straw and had to stand out in the cold rain with the nut running in the wind and rain on the side of I-10. I immediately started telling her what I was doing and how I was supposed to go through Show Low but had to reroute and that's why I was running on the highway. I was talking incredibly fast and I could tell the woman cop was trying to hide a giggle. Turns out, New Mexico doesn't have laws against running on I-10 and had no problem with me running where I was and just stopped to make sure I was okay. After I thanked her, I returned to the head-down running.

CHAPTER 33

Running along the highway in rural New Mexico was very uneventful. I didn't meet anyone for a couple of days, and therefore wasn't able to spread the word of the reason I was running. In those days though, I was able to do a couple of newspaper articles for cities that were close, but not necessarily in driving range, and also did a couple radio interviews. It was really just Grandpa and I, and it was nice getting to know him. The uneventful days were the ones where he and I just hung out and either figured out the route for the next day, or tried to stay on top of the emails that flooded my phone—he was very impressed with the iPhone's capabilities. It was also a time for him to share stories about his life, and the things I never knew about him. We also were able to spend some time scoping other people's trailers because he was in the market for a new trailer at the time. He has since gotten one, but I'm sure it's not quite the same as the Chinook.

Along the side of the road after going through the town of Deming, we saw a winery. I didn't even know there were any wineries in New Mexico. We went in and ordered the tasting special. The first one I just drank for lack of knowledge. He just laughed and said, "You're not supposed to chug it."

He then taught me to swirl it in the glass first. Then smell it and try to smell the type of wood of the barrel it was in. Smell it while you swirl it. Then look at the lines on the glass that the wine leaves behind. The more lines there are, the higher the alcohol content of the wine. Once you take a small sip, hold it on your tongue for a little bit tasting the subtleties in the different wines.

I appreciated him telling me, but to be honest, I don't spend a whole lot of time licking trees, so my tongue wasn't highly trained to taste the difference between the different woods the barrels were made of. I am, however, trained in the fine art of eating loads of chocolate, so when it came to tasting the dessert chocolate wine, I was all for it and my keen senses picked it up immediately.

Toward the end of the series of "mindless" days, I was running along a particularly straight stretch of road next to train tracks and I really hoped a train would come by so I could feel the earth shake as it rumbled next to me. Usually, I didn't like looking backwards while I was running. It often felt like I hadn't come very far and I wasn't getting much done.

For whatever reason today, I looked back but instead of seeing the blank barren land and asphalt that I had traveled across and seen for the past few hours, I saw an additional sight. I saw two black dots which appeared to be bicycles heading my way. After a little while the two got closer and I was able to see that their bikes were loaded down with equipment like they had been on the road for awhile, and planned to be for quite awhile longer.

As they rode up behind me, they slowed down and of course we started talking. Walking around in a city and not saying, "Hi" while you pass someone isn't always rude, but out here, where there is no one, it's not so much a factor of not being rude, but more of a "curious why you're out here too" factor. I learned their names were Russ and Laura. They were both sitting down on their bikes, so it was hard to gauge how tall either of them were but neither seemed abnormally short or tall.

Russ was Asian and wore thick rimmed glasses. They say that everyone has a twin somewhere in the world, and I found my friend, Scott's twin that day when I met Russ. He was medium build, and I got the feeling that both were biking to experience the country rather than for speed because neither of them were wearing the standard, "fast-biker skin-tight" apparel. Both had pants on that were rolled at the bottom to avoid getting stuck in their bike chains and somewhat heavy jackets to stay warm.

Laura was lean and had short brown hair cut about the same level as her ears and fair skin. After talking for a minute, I learned that they are biking AROUND the country. They started in British Columbia and are going to be on the road for a total of about a year and a half, but that time frame wasn't definite. They were enjoying themselves, it seemed, and were enjoying being vagabonds.

They rode ahead a bit and stopped at the RV parked on the shoulder of the road. Russ pulled out a camera with a large lens and began snapping pictures of me running toward them. There were no cars to worry about so he was just lying in the middle of the road catching different angles and different light. He was a very good photographer and would do family portraits of some of the people they stayed with. He specializes in portraits, and photographing food, which I know, is sometimes impossible to make something not look like a pile of trash on a plate. We took several pictures and then a couple with Grandpa and we were each on our ways. I liked talking to someone who was also doing something physical while crossing the country at the same time.

One of the highlights of the day was ending my time on I-10. It turned out to be a 35 mile day with the last 11 on the interstate but I ended right near Las Cruces and wouldn't have to run on the interstate anymore which I was very thankful for.

CHAPTER 34

Approaching Las Cruces was kind of exciting. It was like being a cowboy and being out in the sticks for awhile and then coming back to the big city and civilization. Las Cruces sits in a bowl of land. There are mountains on the east side, and the north side. The south goes to El Paso, TX and Mexico, and coming from the west was an all downhill run.

I am always disappointed running through cities though because from far off it looks like a bustling, exciting place of activity, but when I actually get there, it is not much different than every other city. Fast food joints on every corner, sidewalks that are slanted at very odd angles, drivers who could care less about who has the right-of-way, strip malls with all the same stores as every other city and gas stations that make it a bit hard to breathe for a minute or two as you run past them. Las Cruces was no different except there were way more Mexican restaurants than any other kind. I made my way through the city the day after I met Russ and Laura and once again, was disappointed with the city and wished I was running in the mountains I could see nice and clearly now in front of me.

Leaving the very populated part of the city, the road I was on turned into a highway unexpectedly and once again I had to dodge cars and trucks entering and exiting the highway. In front of me I could see the road turn into a skinny strip of black that kept going straight, but made its way straight up the side of the mountain in front of me. I was excited to be climbing something and this made me go a little faster, and a little stronger.

Since it was the end of the day I decided not to stop running and ran the entire hill which turned out to be a lot longer than it looked from the bottom and a lot steeper as well. I was glad I did too because nothing; I say, NOTHING makes you feel more like a man than cruising steadily up a mountain while you listen to semi-trucks struggle up the same slice of road. I ended the day at St. Augustine Pass which had an elevation of 5,719 ft.

The climbing must have made me hungry because that night we ate at IHOP and since they were having the all-you-can-eat-pancakes promotion I decided to see if they'd cut me off. After 2 eggs, 2 sausage links, hash browns and 14 pancakes, I decided I'd had enough and they weren't going to cut me off. The waiter was intrigued at my constant quest for more pancakes and commented, "Man you really put the pancakes away for such a skinny dude." My Grandpa told him what we were doing and after we got talking I learned that I wasn't doing as well in the pancake eating department as I thought I was. There was a guy that came in a week earlier and destroyed 24 pancakes, but he was a little "heftier" as the waiter put it.

We slept in the IHOP parking lot because there was no reason not to.

CHAPTER 35

I woke up the next morning while it was still dark to the sound of Grandpa starting the RV and driving out of the parking lot. I looked up, from my sleeping bag.

"I want to see the sunrise from St. Augustine Pass," he said. I had no opposition to that.

It was very cold at the pass as we waited for the first few rays of sun to expose the east side of the mountains we were standing on. I looked out at the road that seemed to fall down the side of the mountain that I would soon be falling down myself, and ahead at the long stretch of asphalt that I would be crossing over the next two days. The road looked like God had tried to patch a crack in the earth with black electrical tape and the color faded with time. It was so straight, I couldn't comprehend what I would do in that time to keep my mind occupied. The earth looked so big from up there. I could easily understand how they thought the earth was flat back in the day. It didn't even start to curve at the ends of my line of sight.

The earth before us started to turn pink and then darker pink, then red and then orange made its way into the scene. Just as the sun first peeked up from the horizon, it seemed like I could see that it was on fire. It wasn't just a far-away orb; it was on fire, and I could see the flames. While we stood there for a little while we saw how much different the same place looked at the different time of day. The mountain I had climbed yesterday was exposed as sheer rock with far more cracks than I had noticed on the overcast day yesterday had been. The rough terrain looked even more rugged because of the long shadows that every larger bump in the rock cast over the lesser bumps. Pockets of snow that hadn't melted because they sat in the shadows of cracks in the rock speckled the mountain that I gawked at and gave the mountain an even colder, more rugged look.

I would have rather climbed the face of the mountain that was staring back at me than run on straight roads to more nowhere, but that would not advance me toward my end goal of the Atlantic Ocean, so I turned around and looked at the road I'd be heading down in only a few minutes and I was disappointed at how dull it looked. I much preferred climbing that hill than descending because the view going up was so much better than going down.

When I finally did start the run, it turned out not to be so bad. I enjoyed looking out over the land while the bottom half of me rolled down the long hill. It seemed that I was going down for far longer then I ascended the day before, but I didn't question it too much. After the initial descent, it was just as I had thought, straight road with minimal distractions. There is something spectacular about a desert. It amazes me how there can be so much of nothing, and yet, it is something just by virtue of the definition of matter. It's home to all sorts of animals, but it seems to be lifeless. The slight changes in topography have a meaning, and a reason that no one on earth will ever fully be able to explain. Why is this rock in this spot and not another? Maybe an animal moved it, maybe it's been sitting in the same spot for the past million years. Questions can be asked while viewing the blank mess that is the desert, but exact answers will not be answered. I asked myself many questions while going through this part of the desert and none of them were answered by running more miles—nor did I expect them to be. Chances are good that you'll ask the same questions over and over and only get an answer if you supply it.

The straightness of the road was both astounding and mind numbing. There are some things that I'm not sure we, as humans, are supposed to be able to comprehend. Infinity, for instance is one, and the vastness of a desert with nothing between you and the other side of the desert is another. More than 50 miles in the distance was a mountain that was white with snow, and from the looks of the clouds in the area, was becoming whiter. I would be next to that mountain in two days and I looked forward to seeing the 12,000 ft giant up closer.

It was hard to appreciate everything that was going on around me while I was in the desert because my movements felt pointless. That mountain would stay in front of me without getting any noticeable distance closer even after the hours went by. I would pass grains of sand by the millions with every stride, and yet, I could still see the point where I started, and I could see where I would be in two days. It was a treadmill of land just passing under me while the scenery never changed. Tiny brittle shrubs, clearly dehydrated, existed on the side of the road and the only future they had was to become a tumble weed. I asked myself why they were here. I didn't see a single bird eating its crunchy leaves or using it for nesting material. I didn't see any animals using it for a shelter, not that it would be much of one. What would make something grow in sand? It wasn't even holding any sand in place to prevent erosion like the grasses on dunes at the beach do. It just sat there, seemingly serving no purpose to the world. Philosophical questions made me forget I was running that day, but when I stopped thinking I remembered that things hurt on my legs, and so I concentrated on asking myself questions and coming up with answers.

I ask a lot of questions even when I'm not running. I always have. When I was a little kid my parents bought me the "Big Book of Tell Me Why." I asked so many questions, they ended up buying the second "Tell Me Why Book," because I asked too many questions that the first book didn't answer. Things like, "Why is the sun still round if it's on fire?" "What is wind and where does it start?" And one my mom likes to remind me of, "Does fairy dust make birds fly?" I thought of that one after watching Peter Pan. When it comes down to it, I am able to keep my mind occupied quite well.

The day ended at White Sands National Park. Despite the name sounding "green," there was nothing more than a group of buildings that marked the place where they used to test Atomic Bombs and other rockets and space things. It was also near Holloman Airforce Base, so we stayed in the RV park there because Grandpa is Retired Army.

CHAPTER 36

Running toward Alamogordo was an experience to say the least; I could see the town from a long ways away and got slightly frustrated that it wouldn't get closer faster. Once I got to it, though, I turned straight north toward Tularosa. Running on that road was unpleasant due to the number of cars, and the heavy slant of the shoulder of the road. I ran into a biker who was biking across the country. As we approached each other, we slowed but then he said, "I'm really in a hurry. I'm sorry I can't talk longer."

Before he was too far away he yelled back, "Are you running through Ruidoso?"

"Yea!"

"You're going to love it! It's a great run, and it's just where I came from."

That made me look forward to the next couple of days even more where I would be in the mountains.

I walked through the Village of Tularosa so I could see everything and wouldn't miss anything. There were lots of pistachio trees all around, but were barren because of the winter when I saw them. When I got to the ending point there was a family there with the RV and Grandpa. It was the Brillante family I was going to have dinner with the night I ran up to Ruidoso Downs. Little Feliciana had a doctor appointment and saw me running as they were on their way home, so they stopped and talked with us.

The next day was frigid and pouring rain, so I was happy to have an off day scheduled. We hung out in the RV, read our books, and then visited the NASA museum they had in Alamogordo.

We stayed at an RV park that night and while talking with the owners, they offered us a free night's stay as a donation to the run! They were just strangers but were interested in helping me out, and help they did. The pair also contacted the newspaper in Alamogordo and set me up with an interview for the morning of the following day.

CHAPTER 37

The morning started with the newspaper interview that the owners of the RV park set me up with. Following the interview I started my daily skip and was very happy to do so. Not only had the day before been a day off, but I knew today's run would be in the mountains, and I love the mountains. I wasn't completely sure of how long the hills were, or how steep, how high, or how cold they would be, so I decided to take it easy that day. I would just relax, and enjoy the views, the cool, crisp air, and really try to enjoy being in among majestic giants.

The plan worked because soon after I started the day's run, I began climbing. I just kept going up. Every now and then I would pass an elevation sign, and a little part of me would get giddy, and I would feel a little bit stronger. The higher I ran, the more snow surrounded me. Signs cautioning drivers about elk lined the road, and tiny hillside chapels collected snow on their roofs.

The scenery continued as I climbed higher and higher. I entered the Indian reservation and the barriers on the side of the roads were painted with their ancestor's symbols as well as the names of the school on the reservation. Pictures of bears, eagles, elk, and wolves kept me company up the long hills and shallow descents. Every now and then I would pass under an elevated walkway where people could cross the street and not worry about cars slipping on the ice and hitting them.

As I ran closer to one of them I noticed a banner on it. Still too far away to read it, I ran faster thinking that it said, "Patrick" on it. It got clearer, and when I was able to read it, it said, "Run Patrick Run." And it was covered in painted foot prints of kids. The first thing I thought of was, "Wow! This is cool . . . I wonder how much paint got on the carpet after painting little kids' feet . . ." I took several pictures and looked around for someone to thank but I didn't see anyone, so I continued running.

After several hours of running up hill, I stopped at the RV for lunch. The menu was peanut butter and jelly; two because I was very hungry. We questioned how much further the mountains could keep going up considering I had been climbing for about 25 miles at that point. I found it a little funny how much colder my grandpa was than I because of his thin, Southern California blood. It was cold up there, but it wasn't *that* cold. A short break later, I resumed running—up; and after only about 15 more minutes, there it was: the summit. It was called Apache Summit and was at an altitude of 7591 ft. Being the flat-lander I am, that was higher than I had ever been up until that point. Up on top of the mountain, there was a fire department. I thought it was kind of weird except when I thought about it, it made sense. No matter where the fire is, it's a downhill cruise to the scene. After I thought about it, the top of a mountain was the smartest place for a fire department I had ever seen. "No need to lug a giant truck up a mountain, let's put it on top!" I could hear them planning it in my head.

The next 5 miles were downhill. The scenery hadn't changed a bit; beautiful mountains and thick evergreen forests. And it was even easier to see because I wasn't leaning into the mountain. As I started my decent, a 12,000 ft mountain appeared in front of me and I wondered what it would be like to be standing on top of it. I'm sure I'd be waist deep in snow, but still, it had to be incredible up there. I kept on rolling right on down the side of the mountain making sure I wasn't pounding the pavement and was just cruising and rolling. After 5 miles I reached the end of my rationed number of miles. I looked at the map and discovered that the place we were staying was just 5 miles ahead. I felt great, and even fresher than I started, so I decided it'd be easiest from a logistical standpoint to just continue running and then we wouldn't have to drive back up 5 miles tomorrow to start. More downhill and the legs just churned out the miles effortlessly. After I reached the end of the run in the town of Ruidoso Downs I looked around the little town and I liked what I saw.

It was a quiet little mountain town, with a casino right up the road, and a ski resort close by as well. The town had the essentials but nothing extra. It seemed, to me, to be a well planned town where the planners had brought in everything they needed but would keep to the limits of what makes a town intimate and quaint. The people seemed lively yet friendly, busy, but not too busy to say, "Hi," and relaxed, but not sleepy. It seemed like the best combination of "small town America" and "ski village America" without the kinds of people who just came because they were loaded with cash. This place had purpose, and I immediately felt comfortable here. The air was clean and it was a dry cold, not like the humid cold of the east coast. It could've been 15 degrees colder, and felt warmer than the temperature on the east coast. I looked up at the 12,000 foot peak above the town and took a deep breath. I could feel the cold air inflate my lungs and warm even before I had a chance to breathe it out. I was fascinated that I had never heard of this place before. I knew there were trails somewhere on that mountain and all over the wooded area that surrounded the town that were already neglected from being under snow, but come summer time, they would be ready to be romped on properly and I was just the man for the job.

Grandpa and I found the hotel that the family had donated. Just outside we met a man who worked there but wasn't wearing any kind of uniform. He was dressed in jeans and a long sleeve polo shirt. He never told me his name and his name tag was all scratched from years of wear but he was an older Middle Eastern man who had jet-black hair, and a somewhat scraggly beard. He was about 5' 6" and stood very strong and was stocky. The man looked like he could take a punch or two but wouldn't hurt a fly. A perpetual smile spread across his face and the wrinkles that covered the front of his head proved to be the only thing about him that showed any aging. The man had come to the area after being raised in India. He was really funny, and after we got talking for awhile, he asked me what I was doing in Ruidoso Downs. When I told him, he immediately spoke up, "Oh my goodness is there anything else you need?"

I assured him that I appreciated the offer but I was fine, and would be alright.

"Would you like me to turn up the heat on the hot tub? Can I get you some extra coffee? Extra Pillows? Maybe some Advil?" Anything you need to make your stay more comfortable?"

Again, I told him I much appreciated the kind offers, but wouldn't need anything extra while I was there, except maybe a shower and a good night's sleep.

"Well, if you change your mind, and if you think of anything else you need," he stared writing something on a small piece of paper, "you call this number. Day or night." And then he slid me the phone number where I would be able to reach him.

Grandpa and I were able to shower and relax for a bit. I didn't realize how tired I was until I had taken a shower and changed into dry, warm clothes but I lied down and promptly fell asleep. When I awoke, some twenty minutes later, I realized I was going to need a boost before we met up with the family to eat dinner, so I went down to the lobby to get a cup of coffee.

I saw the man I had met before. He saw me going for the coffee and he yelled something to me. I couldn't hear what he said, but before I had time to un-wrap a mug and pour coffee in it, he came scurrying out from the back room with a fresh pot of coffee.

He said, "I made it, just for you, just in case you wanted some coffee after a long run."

The guy had read my mind. We sat in the lobby and talked while we both sipped coffee. He told me about where he had come from and his two sons, and where they were now. I told him about some of the things I had seen in the first month I was on the road. Before I knew it, the whole pot of coffee was gone and it was time to meet up with the family for dinner. I thanked the man and I met back up with Grandpa.

We both went downstairs to meet up with the family and I was able to remember their names this time. There were two kids, Gabby, who skateboarded, and her little sister, Feliciana. Felicie, as her family called her, has JRA and was diagnosed when she was two and a half years old, but you would've never known. She was a bit shy at first, but by the end of dinner was talking up a storm in her cute little, 4 year old voice. Their parents, Jason and Anne, along with extended family all joined us for dinner at the local Mexican restaurant. Being inside a small, warm restaurant, in a large family setting while temperatures outside dropped quickly, was very comfortable. We sat and talked about the area, the run so far, Felicie's battle with the disease, and how much they all loved it there. Listening to how much they liked it, and how great the area was, made me want to stay. After what seemed like minutes, I looked at my watch, and it was getting late so we said our goodbyes and made our way to our hotel room after the kids signed the banner.

The next day greeted me with cool temperatures and air that burned my lungs the first couple times I inhaled. Running on the sidewalk through the rest of the town of Ruidoso Downs, New Mexico I saw the town in the early morning light and ran in and out of the shadows of the huge mountains that surrounded the town.

As I started the run I noticed that I was still running downhill. The decent would continue for the remainder of the day. Toward the outward limit of the town I saw Grandpa giving me the signal to come over to the side of the road. When I got closer to the RV I saw a class of small kids all bundled up in their large coats and their teachers waving to me. I went over to say hi and realized it was Jason's mother, Linda, from dinner last night. She had a class of preschoolers who were holding Gatorade and beef jerky for me. I talked with them while I sipped on Gatorade and took some pictures. After a while, I was on my way downhill again. The scenery was great the whole day and I decided to add an extra few miles because of the effortlessness of the run that day.

We stopped directly at, what looked to be, an RV park behind a little general store. From first glance, there was one RV in the entire park but neither of us thought anything of it. We went into the store to see about staying in the park overnight and a lady walked out from behind the counter. She said, "Hi, can I help you?"

"We were looking for a place to stay for the evening. Can we stay in the RV park?" Grandpa replied.

"Well, actually," she paused for a moment, "the RV park isn't exactly open."

"Really?" Grandpa seemed surprised.

"I'm not exactly in business anymore . . ."

She went on to explain that she just bought the place with the intention of turning it into an RV park and was promised that everything was approved and up to par. But as it turned out, this was far from true. The seller also had sold her a restaurant space with lots of "equipment" but that turned out to be a bust too. She had really invested everything she had in this place and believed it would turn out for the best, but that was before she found out nothing worked. And to make matters worse, she had to be out in a week from when we saw her and she had mountains of stuff to pack but had no idea what to do with it after it was packed.

Nothing was going right for this woman.

At the end of all this, she still said that we were welcome to camp out behind the general store but she wasn't going to charge us because nothing worked.

Neither of us could believe it. This woman who was losing everything could've very easily said that everything worked and it costs $3000 for a night, but instead she charged us nothing.

We were very appreciative, but decided it was best to pay her regardless.

Chapter 38

The couple of days leaving the mountains were somewhat depressing, and mostly flat or rolling hills with large stretches of straight, flat, plain-like landscape. I found it very surprising how quickly the land went from jagged rocks in the form of mountains to rolling, grassy hills, to flat desolation without even so much as a single tree to disrupt the monotony of it all. Once again, without the grandiose mountains and quaint little towns to take my mind of every step I took, it was back to what became known as "zombie running." I would focus on one point in the horizon and not break my stare for several minutes just to see if something would change around me. Or I would stare at the white line passing under my footfalls and not break my concentration on it for awhile hoping that when I finally looked up I would gain a new perspective on the same land I had been looking at.

Every now and then I would pass a skeleton of some small animal that had met his demise on the side of the road and transformed into road kill in the blink of an eye. I would look at the contorted skeleton for a minute and figure out which leg was supposed to be where and whether or not someone had tossed the remains here in that way. Or maybe they had gracefully been hurled to the side of the road by a vehicle that sent them to whatever higher being they believed in.

I liked to think that they died suddenly from the terror of a giant truck rather than being hit by the roaring concoction of rubber and metal. But after looking at the mangled remains, I realized that this probably was not the case. Maybe they were already dead, and vultures and other scavengers did most of the mangling after the animal had passed, or maybe they died of old age and their family members brought them here to the side of the road to rot so the wind from the passing cars would send the stench of the decaying flesh into my nostrils and it wouldn't be around theirs.

I couldn't count all the possibilities I came up with for how the dead animal died and became part of my view on this trip, but thinking of the different ways, occupied my mind for quite awhile and many long runs. Maybe it is a little morbid, but I had to keep my mind from wandering off too much, and dead animals were a good way to do it.

That evening I ran into Roswell, NM and, of course, saw lots of alien themed murals and stores. The McDonalds in town is a giant UFO-looking saucer and the restaurant was inside the main part of the spaceship. Everywhere I looked there was something to do with aliens, and most stores had the same theme.

I stayed with the Sonive family that night and they were a very entertaining bunch. A four member family, the parents were named Dirk and Whitney and their two sons were Mason and Gage. They lived around Roswell and around their house grew pecan groves. I felt a different kind of connection with this family than some of the others I had met and stayed with.

My mom works at an adult activities center for mentally retarded adults and throughout middle school and high school, I would go into her work on some of my days off. I would help feed "her people," as she calls them, and play games with them throughout the day. Sometimes we'd go bowling, or to the local park as well. I enjoyed it because they were just like grown up kids. It was kind of like playing board games with a 5 year old that had to shave. They had great senses of humor and would say some really off-the-wall stuff that would have all the staff laughing. I was able to see what happens to the kids from the special education classes after they graduate high school.

The Sonive's eldest son, Gage, was autistic. It was interesting to see how autism can affect a family and really shape how they do things differently on a day to day basis. Gage loved to take baths so if a door to the bathroom was open, he would go in and take a bath—clothes and all. So, we had to make sure we kept the bathroom doors closed. It sure beats the way I was as a kid. I never wanted to take a bath.

I also found it interesting to see the family side of autism. I saw how staff was with some grown up autistic people but now I was able to see how family life was with autism.

Roswell as a city was also very dusty. Looking over large plains I could see where the wind was picking up because the dust picked up with it. There were also very strong winds that brought with it the smell of cow manure from the surrounding farms. It was a little bit disturbing at first because this was no ordinary cow manure smell, this was a little bit more rotten, but sure enough, after only a few minutes, I had gotten used to it. Grandpa, on the other hand smelled it for a little longer than I did and took quite a few opportunities to talk about it until I, too, smelled it again.

CHAPTER 39

Days were cold now, and there always seemed to be a freezing wind whipping over the increasingly flat land that I continued to cross on foot. If the air ever remained calm for long enough for the sun to reach my face, I'd realize it wasn't all that cold; but that didn't happen very often.

The land became awkward: very flat for long periods of time and then short steep little canyons that someone had done their best to pave over. The hills never really seemed to stop. I liked those sections though, because it gave me a reason to take walking breaks. And the little aches and pains in my legs, and entire body for that matter, would still make guest appearances on a daily basis.

There were an increasing amount of oil wells—large steel rigs that move up and down pumping the black gold from the seemingly dead land. I remember seeing them as a kid when we lived in Monterey, CA while driving to visit my grandparents in Los Angeles. I was just in preschool and I remember thinking that they looked like giant horses moving up and down while eating. I liked my preschooler brain, and how much the steel rigs still reminded me of horses when you look at the ones that are far off in the distance. They smelt like a mixture of oil and old cow manure. I couldn't tell if there was a lot of manure in the fields they were placed in, or whether that was just the smell that was produced by the pumps. I was expecting it to smell a bit like a gas station, but the two smells are far from similar.

Leaving Roswell meant that I would be in Texas very soon. Texas seemed to be a big goal to reach when I started, and now I would be standing at the border about to start across one of our country's largest states. I was excited to feel like I was making progress and about to cross another one of the eight states off my list.

It was also a bit disheartening to think that soon Grandpa would be heading back to his home and I would really be doing this on my own for the rest of the trip. We had seen cold days, pouring rain, and lots of snow. I'm not sure I could handle all those elements on my own and not hurt myself in some way. It was nice to know that within 5 miles at all times was someone I could call if a freak accident happened. I had a set of wheels that had a motor on it if I absolutely needed to get somewhere, or even if we just needed food and didn't "feel" like walking. I also had a roof over my head every night. If someone offered for us to stay there, sure, it was nice and highly appreciated, but if no one offered and we were in the boonies, we would still have a roof over our heads. All of the "what-ifs" supplied my brain with questions of what I would do in certain situations, but I didn't want to put any pressure on Grandpa to stay any longer—he had a life to get back to.

Before I ran into Texas I had one more off day with the RV. We were in Tatum, NM. The local postmaster, Sandy, helped my family a great deal with delivering a package to me. My dad contacted her about how to send a package to her at the post office in Tatum and hold it until I picked it up. They had been corresponding back and forth for about a week before I got there, I know because I was copied on all the emails—and there were lots of them.

When I walked in, she looked at me and said, "I know who you are!" and went over and got a big box off of the shelf. We talked for a bit about how the run had been going so far and took a picture for the website. She was very kind and really helped us out so that I would receive that box.

When we got back in the RV, I tore into the box. In it, I found a note from my mom, a running magazine, a book, candy, and bags of home-made bird nest cookies.

Let me take a minute to explain the intricacies of my mom's famous bird nest cookies. First you make peanut butter cookie-dough. Roll it into balls and place on a cookie sheet. Bake for awhile, and when you take them out, while they are still soft poke the top with a fork to make a little cavern and drop a few semi-sweet chocolate chips in there. They will start to melt and will later harden into this awesome ball of chocolate peanut buttery goodness; soft cookie, slightly harder chocolate. Perfect.

Eating them is a whole other art in itself. There is what I like to call the "Nest Robber," where you eat the chocolate out of the center first, and then eat the peanut butter cookie part separately. Next is the, "Cement Mixer," where you bite the cookie in half and the mixture of chocolate and peanut butter mix beautifully in your palate—much like a cement mixer. The final method of eating the bird nest cookie is called, "The Kevin," named after my little brother. The way to achieve "The Kevin" is to shove at least three of the cookies in your mouth at the same time without choking. While slightly risky, this method will ensure the maximum amount of fun for those watching you, and will also be difficult to do without choking. If you do start to choke, which you will, bend at the waist, look at the ground, close your eyes, and swing your head violently so cookie flies out of your mouth and all over all of those that made fun of you.

Anyway, the famed bird nest cookies had been in the mail for a whole week, but they were still soft and very delicious. I stuck to the first and second method of eating them to be sure that I didn't waste a single crumb of this beloved cookie.

CHAPTER 40

Following the day off, I started my run into Texas. Fueled by bird nest cookies, I trucked along in the cold wind. It even started to snow a little bit. It was a very low day for me. I remember it being especially low because I didn't know anything about what would happen even that night. There was so much unknown and I couldn't stop thinking about it.

After running for awhile on the flat New Mexican land, I saw a sign that said something about a Caprock. I didn't know anything about it, and didn't really care. I went up a steadily inclining road and then it leveled off after another little while. I gave it no thought and kept right on going. Lots of cattle were out in the cold grazing and getting covered in the increasingly heavy snow. And they ran away when I got close. I thought I could feel the ground move when some of the larger ones ran. The snow came down in small flakes, but there were lots of them, and none that stuck to the ground. They melted on my mittens and so I kept my hands balled up in fists to keep my fingers from going completely numb. I got lots of strange looks while I was running along the side of a road in the middle of nowhere, while it was snowing, and wearing running shorts. I wore a hat to keep my head covered, a long sleeve running shirt, SmartWool sweater, and a Buff to keep my nose from freezing.

I passed the sign welcoming travelers to Texas, took some pictures, and took a lunch break. I realized this would be the last time I could sit down mid-day and make my own peanut butter and jelly sandwiches while I warmed my extremities in a cave on wheels. After I resumed running, it warmed up nicely, and the snow stopped, the sun came out and it became a very pleasant day. As I ran into Plains, Texas I saw Grandpa up ahead parked in a motel parking lot. He said he heard there was going to be snow that night so he would get me a room instead of leaving me to fend for myself in the snow.

Taking the stroller off of the bike rack on the front of the RV, and cleaning out my supplies wasn't fun. I started to get rather nervous and didn't want him to leave. The room wasn't quite 5-star, but it wasn't terrible. I didn't really care about staying in sketchy hotels, but the fact that I was saying goodbye to Grandpa and staying in a room with a heater that had to be lit with a lighter added to the decreased spirits. When all of my supplies were in the room and accounted for, there was nothing else to do but say goodbye to the one person I hadn't said goodbye to in Huntington Beach. I thanked him for coming with me and doing such a great job accompanying and supporting me, and then said, "Drive safe," hugged him and parted ways. I closed the door and could feel myself start to cry. I had become increasingly bad at goodbyes on this trip, especially to those who had become my life-line for so long.

During that evening I packed up my stroller. I also made my "tower of peanut butter and jelly" that would become a vital part of my calorie intake for the vast majority of the days that I spent on the road. I had a whole loaf of bread, and a jar of peanut butter, and a small jar of jelly. I made all of the sandwiches for the whole loaf and used the whole jar of jelly so I didn't have to carry that with me anymore. Then I stacked the sandwiches and put them back in the bread bag so it looked like a loaf of bread.

I sat by the "live fire" heater and read that night but couldn't really focus on the story. I was reading about 23 year old Bear Grylls climbing Mount Everest. I was too busy thinking about how much different the trip would be without Grandpa. The next day would be the first day of uncertainty for me when I got to the next town 35 miles away. The towns in west Texas along the road I was running were strategically placed about 25-35 miles apart. Perfect for a starting and ending point, but if something went wrong in the middle, I wouldn't know how to deal with that. With the barren land came a loss of cell coverage, at no fault of the cell phone companies, but because of the lack of people.

CHAPTER 41

I awoke the next morning to the alarm clock and the heater warming the left side of my face. The right side seemed extremely cold, and I could only guess how cold it would be outside. Looking toward the curtain-covered window in the room, I could see the illumination of something bright lighting the edges of the curtains. I pulled the curtain aside to see what it could be. I was greeted by the sight that as a kid I dreamed of every school day of the year: snow.

There was a good 3 inches on the ground already and it was still coming down. I pulled on all the gear I had packed for the outside chance this would happen and started down the road heading east. Luckily it was a very wet snow and didn't stick very well to the road. Mostly the roads were just wet, but even the areas that did accumulate some snow were easy for the tires of the baby jogger to cut through.

The wind whipped the snow around me and the jogger in a mini tornado of flurries. I got that giddy feeling of being outside while it was snowing and *enduring* more. Cars were moving very slowly and cautiously through the town, which I appreciated greatly because visibility was low. I had attached some blinking red lights to the front of the jogger, wore a reflective belt, and wore a headlamp just to be on the safe side.

It didn't take long to get out of the town of Plains, Texas and when I did there was nothing but flat farmland that looked to be hibernating. Covered in a soft blanket of snow the fields looked depressed. I knew that during the warmer months this land was lively with crops, but now, the old dead stalks, still in their rows that went on forever, were the only thing poking through the snow. A car pulled up slowly going the same direction I was and asked if I needed a ride.

"Need a ride?" The man spoke hesitantly like this was not the first question he wanted to ask me.

"No thank you, but I really appreciate the offer."

"But . . . the next town is more than 30 miles away!"

"Thanks for the heads up, but I have to run it. I'm raising money for juvenile arthritis." I handed the man one of my cards.

" . . . Okay son, good luck."

"Thanks again!"

The guy looked at me like I was a nut case as he drove off.

I would get 5 more ride offers that day and each one would be a little bit harder to turn down. Because it was still snowing, I was getting a bit wet. The rain jacket and rain pants that I had gotten for the trip were, I thought, water proof, but after that day I realized they were just water resistant. I gradually got more and more wet, and more and more cold. I was able to stay warm as long as I was running, but if I stopped for any reason, I immediately started to feel the cold; so I kept running.

The snow would ease up here and there for one minute, or 15, only to start again without fail.

As I entered the town of Brownsfield I called the mayor of Post, Texas due to confusion on my part. My dad had contacted Thressa several days prior because I would soon be running through Post and we wanted the town to be aware of my arrival in case the run and the cause could get any publicity, and also to hopefully find a place to stay in town. There had been many emails flying back and forth, and she mentioned that she might know someone in other towns in west Texas. For whatever reason, I thought she lived in Brownsfield so I called her. After only a minute, I realized my mistake and realized I was in a town covered in 5" of snow and no place to stay. She said she would make some calls and to "hang tight." I surprisingly found a Burger King in the town and went inside to warm up and hopefully get dry. I hung out in there looking like a creep in my soaking wet jacket and pants and my shoes made a squishy noise when I walked because they were full of water.

After some time, I got a call from Thressa saying that she found me a place to stay and a guy would call to give me some details. So, I waited a bit more and did some more people watching. I didn't mind sitting there; I like people watching, and their reaction to seeing the loaded baby jogger outside covered in the orange rain cover. Besides, if I wasn't just sitting there, I would've just been sitting somewhere else, so it was nice to have some built-in entertainment.

After a while longer, a man named Don called me. He asked where I was and said he would be able to get me a room at the local motel. I was incredibly excited and made arrangements to meet him. When I met him, the older man with white hair that stuck out of all sides of the hat he was wearing, smiled very wide and introduced himself. He wrote me a voucher for the hotel and pointed out where it was. He didn't stay long, but I was very appreciative of him giving me a place to stay.

I walked over to the hotel in sweet anticipation of taking off my freezing wet clothes and taking a hot shower and crawling in a warm bed. After checking in I grabbed a newspaper so that I could stuff the paper in my shoes so they would dry overnight. This is an old trick my friend Adam showed me from his days running for the cross country team for our high school.

I'm not sure the door was all the way closed before I began taking off my jacket so I could take a shower. Few things in life are as comforting as taking a hot shower after being out in the cold snow all day, and yet I think it had been something I had taken for granted many times. After I was warm, and my hands were all wrinkled from the water, I got out and began the process of laying all my clothes, supplies, and shoes out to dry. Luckily for me, the clothes were dry by the next day and I was able to pack them without starting a science fair project in my dirty laundry bag.

CHAPTER 42

It was clear the next day and had no snow. It was warmer so much of the snow had melted or was in the process of melting. This made the roads wet, and it looked like it would be another day with wet feet. But as the hours rolled by, the soft breeze seemed to dry everything very efficiently and I didn't have any problems.

The country revealed itself as a dry, barren looking, very dusty place. There were driveways every couple miles that had big signs labeling the driveway as an entry to someone's ranch. But the length of the driveway exceeded the distance of my view because I never saw a single house.

The day turned out to be a day of animals because I saw bison, horses, cattle and prairie dogs. I had never seen bison or prairie dogs outside of the zoo so I found it to be interesting watching the little rodents zip from hole in the ground to hole in the ground. They made a funny screaming noise and I couldn't tell if they were screaming at me or the hawk that circled overhead.

When I reached the town of Tahoka, I went into the gas station to get myself chocolate milk, a chili-dog, a corndog and a doughnut. It was a meal of champions but as I turned to leave the store, a lady looked at me and said, "Oh my God, you're Patrick McGlade." I must admit, I've been confused many times in my life, but that topped it all. I turned around and said, "Excuse me?"

"Aren't you the kid who's running across the country?"

"Yes, how do you know who I am?" I was still incredibly shocked that she knew my name.

"I saw a news segment on you back in January that said you were leaving Huntington Beach."

I was still confused on how she saw a news segment from California in Texas.

"Our station tends to pick up more news from around the country than most news stations. I guess it's because there's not a ton of news in Tahoka."

We talked for a bit outside the gas station about how the run was going so far and what I had seen. I enjoyed the sunny weather and the mid 60's temperature. Her little girl signed my banner and then we parted ways.

I was told through an email that the mayor, John, and his friends Tammi and Michael had gotten me a room at the local motel. They apologized for not letting me stay at their house but they had no room due to current house guests. I assured them it wasn't a problem.

As I was undressing to take a shower I tossed my shoes on the floor, just as I always do, and did the same thing with my socks except they didn't flop the way I expected them to.

It was the most intriguingly cool and mysteriously disgusting thing to grace my eyes in quite some time. Sitting up, in perfect form, right there on the floor were my socks. Standing on their own. I only thought one thing, "Get the camera before the things walk out the door by themselves."

Luckily I was swift with the camera work and was able to document the memorial to sheer dirtiness. The great thing is that even thought they were being held up by a wonderful concoction of dirt, mud, sweat, general road grime, and possibly blood from a cut on my leg, the wondrous SmartWool socks did not smell.

Right near the motel was George's Restaurant, so I grabbed a few hamburgers and a few sides and went back to the room to watch the Olympics opening ceremonies.

CHAPTER 43

Following the day of the dirty, when I found my socks could stand by themselves, was an even warmer day. I ran the straight, flat roads in nothing but shorts and couldn't believe that only two days ago I was running in a small snow storm. I passed lots of ranch driveways, again, with no view of the homes. Toward the end of the day I started running downhill. I thought it was a bit strange but didn't mind it too much. I found it funny that I just kept running down because I couldn't see the bottom of the hill, but I could see the town of Post, TX down below me. After about 15 minutes of running down I reached the bottom of the hill and the town of Post. I didn't know it at the time, but I had just left the Caprock. The same Caprock that I climbed up the day Grandpa left. It is literally just a giant slab of elevated rock, referred to as the Caprock.

I called the mayor, Thressa, and we met up. She showed me a sign that they have in town that welcomed people to Post, and it had my name scrolling across the bottom of it. It was pretty cool to see my name on the sign. She then showed me all around her town and brought me to Holly's Drive-In for a famous burger. I can see why it's famous.

We went to her house so that I could get cleaned up before we went to the local middle school's basketball game. When she showed me her house, she gave me the tour and said, "But you'll be staying out in the shed."

What I found was no standard shed. The outside looked like a normal shed; nice, but not anything fancy. Inside though was a different story. It was themed like a hunting cabin without excessive dead things on the walls. There was a huge bed that looked so soft I would sink into it and sleep on cloud stuffing. There was a bathroom in there with running water, and a TV, and a dresser with a giant mirror on it. Sitting on the bed was a basket she had made with candy, fruit, nuts, and other food. She showed me the fridge and said, "I wasn't sure what you liked, so I put a bit of everything in there."

She wasn't kidding. There was water and Gatorade, Coca Cola Classic, and Diet Coke, Dr. Pepper and Sprite. Then she showed me what I had for breakfast the next morning. It was a whole platter of hardboiled eggs and fruit! She had gone way above and beyond in helping me feel comfortable.

Arriving at the basketball courts, I realized this was an every-kid-in-town kind of event. Anyone who played basketball was here, and everyone knew everyone. I found it interesting that the kids' coaches wore cowboy hats and boots, even on the court. I had heard that people in Texas wore cowboy hats but I can't say I believed them until I saw how many people did.

Afterward, we had dinner with the judge and his wife. They were very nice people and we got into a discussion about what I was *packing* while running. A bit confused, I asked them what they meant.

"What are you packing? What kind of piece do you carry?" They all confirmed the question with nods.

"Like a gun? I don't carry a gun."

They were all a bit surprised I didn't have a gun with me while I was running and then they showed me what a concealed weapons license looked like. Not everyone in Texas is a cowboy, but there are a large amount of people there that still raise cattle, and carry guns. I liked it.

CHAPTER 44

In talking with the Judge of Post, TX, I was able to find someone who would let me stay inside the community center in the town of Clairemont. I was supposed to meet him at 3 o'clock so that he could unlock the building for me after my 27 mile day. I left in time to get there at about 1:30 at my normal pace. I started at about 9:30 am.

The weather decided to keep things interesting for me that day. When I started it was about 65 degrees and sunny with a light breeze in my face. After about 40 minutes the sky darkened, the temperature dropped and the breeze turned into gale force winds that made it impossible to run. I immediately put my shirt on as well as a long sleeve shirt. The date was February 14, Valentines Day, and clearly, someone must have hated me that day because it was miserable. The terrain became incredibly hilly, thus adding to the difficulty of the run, but to my surprise, going uphill provided no shelter from the head on, strong, steady wind, and gravity didn't seem to help me at all on the down hills.

I became incredibly cold and couldn't feel my fingers anymore so I unpacked my entire bag and put on every article of clothing I had. I even put on pants, which usually doesn't even happen if it's snowing. I was having an absolutely miserable day. The wind never let up for one second.

The temperature seemed to drop steadily throughout the day and I was hunted by a hungry dog. He ran up to me barking, snarling, and growling and I ran to the other side of my jogger. I was careful to keep the jogger between the demon dog and me. I saw a man about 50 yards away just watching the hunt unfold. Finally, the owner came up and started beating the crap out of his dog.

He then proceeded to yell at me, "Why didn't you just hit him!?"

"I'm not going to beat your dog! Are you kidding me!?" I was mad at this point. The man continued.

"How else are you going to get a dog to do what you want? You just spent five minutes running around your stroller like a lunatic avoiding a pissed off dog!"

"Maybe if you didn't piss off your dog by beating him, he would've taken to me a little better! You were just standing there just watching me be hunted by your dog!" Clearly, I was not getting through to the man because he continued to scream and yell at me all while clutching the scruff of his snarling dog's neck. I just walked away.

I thought it couldn't get any worse. As 2:30 approached, I expected to see the town soon, but didn't. I checked my phone, but of course, had no signal. 3:00 came and passed, 3:30, 4:00 both passed with no sign of the town. I did my best to get there as soon as I could but the wind was so strong directly into the stroller and my body, all of my effort toward running only produced a modest pace.

After a long time of no cars, a truck pulled up and asked me if I was Patrick. I assured him I was and he introduced himself as the man that would let me into the building. I apologized for not being there on time but he understood considering the weather. He agreed to go ahead and unlock it for me now and told me which door would be unlocked. I asked him for an estimate for how much further it was to the building. He didn't know for sure, but he said it was still quite a ways away. He offered me a ride, but I had to decline the incredibly tempting offer. After I thanked him for helping me, he went ahead to unlock the door to where I'd be staying.

" . . . Quite a ways away . . ." What did that mean? Did he mean by car or on foot? Was he a runner? Was he taking into account how long I'd already been running, albeit, a slow pace? These questions further sunk my already low morale and the rest of the day dragged on and on and on.

It turned into a race against the sun. Having no cell coverage meant I couldn't tell how much longer I had or how long I had already gone. I was a clueless, low, tired, cold runner who wasn't even running. I reached the top of a very long hill and was able to see for miles ahead of me and still didn't see any towns. Starting down the hill there was a huge gust of wind and I got so frustrated I shoved my stroller as hard as I could down the hill. It went about

6 feet, stopped and rolled back up the hill toward me. It was evident; this was the worst day ever.

As I came around a corner at 6:00 pm I saw a sign, "Welcome to Clairmont." There were still no buildings in sight but there were two abandoned houses on my right, and one house with lots and lots and lots of hunting gear surrounding the yard filled with cars. As I continued walking through Clairemont I saw a big building with what looked like a giant barn attached to it. Due to lack of anything else around, I assumed this must be the community center and decided to check the doors. Sure enough I found one unlocked and went inside. It was used during cattle sales as a multipurpose facility. I was happy just to get away from the intense wind, and was pleased that I wouldn't have to set up a tent in such intense conditions. I was incredibly thankful for being able to stay in a building that night. Cell service was spotty at best, but after several attempts it was able to find out that the day that was supposed to be 27 miles turned out to be 38. I was so exhausted by 7 o'clock that I ate a PB and J and as soon as I set up my sleeping bag, I was asleep.

CHAPTER 45

Waking up without an alarm the next day, I packed up and went outside hoping today's conditions would be better. The sun hit my face first, and it felt great even though it was very cold out. Since yesterday had been lengthened, today would be shorter in order to stay on track.

I arrived in Jayton, population 513, around 11:10 am on President's Day; which was strange because it happened to be the day after Valentine's Day that year. Being a holiday, everything was closed; everything except for Sassy's Café. The restaurant was only open from 11-2 that day but I got there just in time. I parked my stroller out front and went inside with my book. I planned on staying inside as long as I could because it was so cold. Then I would find the police station and see if they would let me camp out behind their station. The second I walked, in the sweet aroma of fresh baked goods filled my nostrils and the heat from the heater warmed my face. It felt amazing walking in there and I immediately started thawing out.

I sat down and a lady who was standing next to the heater asked me if I'd like something to drink. She recommended the sweet tea, so I went with that. I hadn't been a huge fan of sweet tea, but it sounded good, so I ordered it. Since I had that tea at Sassy's, I have become a sweet tea enthusiast. I ordered the meatball sub and it was absolutely amazing. I got talking to the lady in there and learned that her name was Deb.

Deb was a short, thin woman with short, brown hair. I could tell she didn't like the cold because she had her arms crossed like she was cold the whole time I was talking to her, and I didn't get the feeling it was because she was angry with me. She spoke with a deep drawl that gave away the fact that she was born in Texas, raised in Texas, and would happily remain in Texas.

"Whatcha doin with that buggy?" She asked.

I told her what I was doing with it. At first, she laughed, "That sounds exactly like something my son would do. You even look like him, just a little bit smaller."

After we got talking for awhile, she asked where I was staying. When I told her I planned on finding a place to camp, she offered her son's room to me. A warm place to sleep? A hot meal? How could I possibly turn that down?

It was also incredibly lucky that she lived on the exact road I would be running on, so I didn't do any extra running! Excited about finding a place to stay through just talking with someone for about 10 minutes, I ran to her house where I was able to take a hot shower and put on clean clothes, something I was unable to do the previous night.

While sitting on the couch, waiting for her daughter to finish school, Deb quickly got up and went to the window facing an air strip across the street from her house. She said,

"You smell that?"

As far as I could remember, in the past five minutes I hadn't let anything loose from the ol' fart cannon, so I replied with, "No, what is it?" hoping I hadn't let one rip without knowing.

"It's smoke."

She ran to get her binoculars from a cupboard and went outside on her porch and looked through them carefully scanning the horizon.

"There it is. It's right over there." And she handed me the binoculars.

I scanned for a minute, and then saw some faint grey smoke rising up in the distance.

"Whoa, there it is. What's on fire?"

"I don't know, but I'm going to call the department."

She picked up the phone and dialed the number by heart even though it wasn't 911. When the man on the other line picked up, she called him by his first name and reported the smoke sighting. I could hear him on the other side of the phone but not clearly. Deb answered him in complete sentences so I was able to easily guess what he asked her.

"Yes, I can see the smoke."

She paused for another minute and then answered him slightly sarcastically the way you would answer an old friend admitting something you weren't really supposed to be doing.

"Yes, I was looking through my binoculars again . . . but I'm serious, there is smoke."

Another pause, and then, "yes . . . okay . . . . thank you." And then she hung up.

She walked back toward the window, and said, "I love my binoculars." I just smiled. I liked the small town feel I had experienced so far.

Deb's husband, Harold, got home after a little while and I was glad I got to meet him. He was a very interesting guy. He was an employee of Mobile Oil, and a collector of old tools. He had light hair and a giant, majestic mustache. He was about 6' 4" and was thin, but rugged. He walked slowly, but with heavy feet in the house, and his size was somewhat intimidating even though he was an incredibly kind man. He showed me his collection of old tools as well as where he kept his garden when the weather got warmer. It was a large area along the right side of their house and he told me what he grew in each row. The shed that he kept all of his tools in could best be described as a proper "man cave." He had everything any man would need to survive out there and also collected Mobile Oil memorabilia because he had worked for them for so long.

In the afternoon he went out to chop some wood and when he got back he had a large oil drum in the back of his truck. He came into the house and insisted we all come outside to look at the large, old, grey drum. I was very surprised that it wasn't rusted, but then again, things don't rust very easily when there is almost no moisture in the air. On one end it said, "Magnolia" on it. Harold said, "They don't make 'em like this anymore. This one is a different size and it says Magnolia on it."

I still didn't see the big excitement over an oil drum. He went on to explain how old it was and that Magnolia became Mobile back in the late 50s. I was starting to see why the man was so stoked on it. For someone who collects Mobile Oil memorabilia, this thing was the king of antiques, the mother lode, and he just found it. We put it in the man cave so no one would steal it. I guess there were a lot of people in the area who collected oil memorabilia.

Their daughter, Denise, had a basketball game that night, so I was able to see two basketball games in three days. They knew everyone in the town, and everyone knew them. I was able to meet many people at the game and tell a lot of people about juvenile arthritis as well as the run.

The next morning I woke up and got ready to head on to the next town. Denise had school that day and Deb asked if Denise would mind if I came to talk to her school. I didn't know about it, until I was talking with Deb and she got a phone call from Denise's teacher asking if I could come into the class. I had no objections so I went in to talk to Jayton Girard School.

Again, I was surprised at the behavior by the students. I expected at least one kid to start acting up, or fall asleep. I think part of me was hoping for an unruly kid because then I'd be able to pelt a piece of chalk or an eraser at them. I think I may have heard too many horror stories from my dad's Catholic school days. But alas, no chalk pelting today, all of the kids were well behaved and again, asked very interesting questions. I was noticing a trend among the middle school age group of students. Many of them were very concerned with where I was going to the bathroom out there.

After meeting with the class, I ran to Aspermont.

CHAPTER 46

Aspermont, at first glance, looks like a town that was resurrected as a place for farmers and ranchers to meet. Most of the businesses in town were stores that benefited that group of people. They had everything from feed stores to tractor repair. There were also some other small shops, but for the most part, it was farming and ranching.

I knew that I was staying with a couple by the name of Jeff and Patti that night, so I went to the high school where Patti worked to meet up with her. Both Patti and Jeff were very kind people. When we got to their house I was able to shower and get clean after a long day's run. Jeff is a preacher for their local church and asked if I would mind going to the basketball game for the high school girls that night. They were in the finals and this game was a big deal for the town and they, as the preacher and his wife, felt it their duty to support the local team. I could tell they just really wanted to go, and I had no problem with that at all. It's a good thing I like watching live sporting events, no matter what age or level of game they are playing.

On the way to the game we saw tons and tons of wind mills on top of a plateau. Apparently, that was a place that always had wind. There were mills as far as I could see.

At the game I met some of Jeff and Patti's friends. One of them was a high school teacher in the town of Rule, a town I would be passing through during my run the following day. She asked if I could come to the school and talk to the seniors. I had never talked to a high school class before, but I didn't think it could be that different, so I agreed.

I ran to Rule as planned, and noticed that it was my halfway point on my way to Haskell, where I would stay that night in a hotel room donated by Vicky from Texas. When I got there, they had a Subway sandwich for me and it tasted delicious. I was still consuming a very large amount of calories per day and working very hard on keeping my body intact. Eating large amounts of food was the best way I knew how to do this, around 6000-8000 calories per day to be exact.

Talking to the seniors was like no speaking engagement I had experienced before. It was so much more relaxed and it felt like I was just telling a group of friends about the stuff I'd been doing lately and why I was doing it. They all sat around their computer lab, and I sat in front of them. There were about 20 or so students all together and I wasn't too much older than them. They weren't any different than I was, young people growing up, trying to figure out what was going on and figuring out how not to appear clueless 95% of the time.

When I spoke with the younger classes it felt like a speaking engagement. I tried to put things in terms the kids would understand, and reference things in their lives they could relate to. Talking to the seniors was easy; I just told it like it was. They were able to understand the awful disease that juvenile arthritis is. They understood what a calorie is and asked questions other than where I went to the bathroom. In a sense, it was nice talking to them, and I really enjoyed it. I believe after talking to them, I wasn't afraid of public speaking anymore. They completely relaxed me, and taught me that talking in front of people no matter the age could feel completely natural and not awkward at all.

Leaving Rule, I ran strong. Fueled by a fresh sandwich, and some Gatorade, I felt good. Physically, I was fueled and ready to tear up the road. Mentally, I felt like I could talk to anyone. I wasn't afraid of people and realized that people were interested in what I had to say, so I should say it more. People are more likely to listen to you telling them about kids with a disease if you believe in it enough to convey that passion. I was stoked enough on telling people about kids with JRA that I was willing to run across the country telling people as I met them. And it took me all the way to Texas to realize that people were going to listen if I told them. I took note of my heightened sense of mentality and ran stronger because of it. I felt fluid and smooth and like I could run straight into the Atlantic from here, but of course, I had to stop for the night, so I stopped at my scheduled stopping point in Haskell.

There was something I noticed going on with my body. It wasn't a change, but it was a craving. I craved fresh fruit and fresh veggies. My body screamed for them.

I would feel terrible if I ate fast food. My stomach would hurt, my intestines would twist, and I would end up a twisted cramped mess. The problem was that I would have to eat 3 or 4 salads from anywhere I'd order them in order to fulfill my calories and appetite. Across from the hotel I was staying at, was a Dairy Queen. I needed food, so I went there because everywhere else was on the other side of town and once I got cleaned up, my desire to go on a hike had diminished. I went there and ordered a stack of salads and a small sundae. It tasted like heaven. It's like my body thanked me even after ordering it before I took the first bite. The vitamins and nutrients in the vegetables seemed to call my name and their voice was sweet. I enjoyed every one of those 5 salads with romaine lettuce, tomatoes, onions, and green peppers with a bit of Italian dressing. And the sundae for dessert was nice to top it all off . . . even though the salads were from a fast food place

The next day was a day off and was spent relaxing, and reading in the hotel room. I did some maintenance on the jogger because the right wheel kept falling off. The jogger always turned left, which started out as a really annoying part of pushing the thing, but after a while, I just got used to it and every couple steps would correct its direction and it became second nature.

I looked at the problem several times and tried to fix it but it turned out to be a miscalculation on the welding in the factory and the two arms that were the fork were uneven. Therefore: it always turned left. Because of the torque of the stroller always turning, the right wheel kept sliding off because the locking mechanism wouldn't lock because it had so much dust and dirt in it from being on the back of the RV for so long. I spent much of the day trying to get the wheel to lock in place so I wouldn't have to keep pushing the wheel back on every half mile or so. The good news is that I was able to fix the wheel; the fork was a lost cause.

I was glad to be able to fix at least one problem on the stroller. Since this stroller was like a form of secondary legs, I needed it to function just like my own legs. Fixing it gave me a sense of relief like I was going to be able to handle bigger problems as they arose.

The hotel room the second night was donated by Jeff and Patti's friend, Tom. I never got to meet Tom, yet, he wanted to help with the run. It was easy to thank the people I met in person for all that they had done for me whether it was a place to stay or a donation to the cause. It was slightly more difficult to truly thank the people who helped me who I had never met and probably wouldn't get the opportunity to meet.

These were the people that I was most surprised about. They didn't know me, they didn't see what I was doing or who I was doing it for, and yet, they still wanted to help. They still wanted to give what they had to someone who needed it. People want to help.

I am still amazed at the amount of people that helped me without meeting me.

CHAPTER 47

Leaving Haskell was a welcomed day. It was a nice town, but any time I took a day off I felt no progression, and therefore got very antsy. I was more than ready to start running again. I wasn't just excited about the sheer fact that I was running that day. That was also the day that I would cross my halfway point.

Halfway across the United States of America. I was thrilled. The run had some great scenery that day; land that extended in every direction as far as the eye could see. There were slow rolling hills that kept the black asphalt somewhat interesting. And every now and then there was a small area of bushes that were native to the area but a kind that I had never seen. I did find it interesting that the days where I felt good mentally, I viewed the empty land as beautiful landscape and found it fascinating that I could see so far without being interrupted by trees, or buildings. The days where I was feeling low, it was boring, and I wanted a different view or anything to take my mind off the mundane task at hand. Today, however, I was in paradise.

It was cold that morning. I started with my mittens on but couldn't decide whether they should stay on or come off. Every time I put them on, my hands would get hot. Then I took them off and my fingers would turn into little frozen sausages. Hot. Cold. Hot. Cold . . .

I checked my phone where I had all my maps. I had one mile until the halfway point. I ran a little more, checked again; I really didn't want to miss this. I went a little further and checked again.

I was on it.

I had run 1,276.5 miles so far, and had 1,276.5 to go. I was on the spot that meant I was halfway across the country in terms of mileage, granted I didn't get lost on the rest of the trip. I did a little dance, made a haunting video of said dance, and then I kept running.

Quite honestly, I thought the high of being halfway would have lasted a bit longer, but thoughts of how cool it was quickly turned to how much further I had. I started thinking about the whole distance and got discouraged. Discourage turned to disappointment, and that brought the mood down quickly. The area around me changed from great scenery to mundane terrain. I tried to focus on the present and to soak it all in so that I would be able to look back on this time at the end and think of what a great time I had, but nothing brought the mood up. I ran into Throckmorton feeling disheveled and disheartened. Martha, who I would meet later, from the Arthritis Foundation, donated the hotel room that night. I was very thankful I was able to shower.

I found a little restaurant that was only open for dinner and went in there with a book to read. People tend to look at you a little bit funny when you're sitting in a restaurant by yourself reading a book wearing running shorts, running shoes and a sweater. I used the time not to read but to catch up on my people watching. I always enjoy watching people. Not to sound creepy, but it's very entertaining; besides, it's not like I follow them home or anything like that. Mannerisms are a funny thing, and they can be the difference between an initial impression of someone being nice, or something other than nice. I also like to watch people having dinner and try to figure out their relationship. Young couples are my favorite, but middle aged is interesting too. I try to figure out if they are dating, married, or related. Once I get there, I try to guess how long they've been married, or if related, if they are siblings, or cousins.

I was still hanging out watching people and eating dessert very slowly. One couple walked into the restaurant and I immediately knew they were married. Both were wearing wedding rings and were outwardly showing they were together . . . not something that would be going on if this were a "side project," especially in this small town. They were middle aged, 40s or 50s, and the guy shot a look my way. *Caught, bummer.* I resumed "reading" and then looked up again only to see the guy still looking at me.

"Hey! Were you running on the road a few miles back today pushing a baby?"

I laughed a little bit, but not so much that I would seem pompous.

"Yes, but it wasn't a baby, it was all my stuff."

"Where are you running to?"

"The Atlantic Ocean."

"What the hell would make you do that? Come over here!"

I went and sat down with him and his wife. Their names were Steve and KT I later learned. I told them about the run, why I was doing it, where I started, where I was going, and gave them a business card.

"Well, I'll be. Well hey; did you already pay for your dinner?"

"No, not yet, but I didn't come over here to get someone to pay for my dinner."

He called over the waitress, and I started to say, "You really don't have to . . ."

"Add whatever he had to our bill, please, ma'am."

The waitress agreed and I was somewhat stunned. I had just met this couple 3-5 minutes ago and the Steve just paid for my dinner. *This is insane!* I thought.

I stayed and talked with them for awhile longer, and they asked me lots of questions. I had no problem answering questions, but sort of felt like I was intruding on "date night." So when their food came, I thanked them profusely for dinner and excused myself. Still, somewhat in shock of what just happened, I walked across the street to my hotel room and fell asleep because the next day would be my longest yet in terms of mileage.

CHAPTER 48

Camping is something that I expected to do for most of the nights on the trip, but places to stay kept falling into place for me; and as long as I had a bed available to sleep in, and a shower available to get clean in, I would try my hardest to get there to use them. This was the case when I ran the next day from Throckmorton to Graham.

The Holiday Inn Express, after contacting them, had agreed to give me a complimentary room for the night and I couldn't pass it up. Besides, Holiday Inn Express' have a killer breakfast, and all the coffee you can drink at almost any hour of the day, or night as the case may be. This being said, I would have to run 40 miles to get there, but then would have to cut back on the following day's miles in order to stay on schedule. This was becoming increasingly important due to the amount of people that were talking to and were contributing to the run.

I had been used to 25-35 mile days, but I hadn't yet done a 40 mile day. I wasn't too worried about it because it was a distance I had covered many times before this trip either in races or on training runs and it was relatively easy for me to do this. I hadn't, however, done it the day after running 33 miles.

I woke up early that day so I could start just as daylight broke just in case I needed all the daylight hours. I had sort of psyched myself out with nervousness, because it all went fine and I ran smoothly, and effortlessly. I did, however, add a few new foods to the food diary for the trip. I ate two corn dogs, a Twix bar, and a half liter of chocolate milk while running and didn't spew; and it wasn't like I was holding the puke back either, I just didn't even get the urge to barf. I was both impressed and proud of myself.

I found the Holiday Inn Express with no problems and upon entering the hotel poured myself a cup of coffee and spent the evening in a room with more pillows than anyone should legally be allowed to sleep with: 14. Why anyone could possibly need 14 pillows between two beds is beyond me.

Being that I ran longer the day before meant that I was going to run a shorter amount of miles the next day, so I stayed in the hotel as long as possible. I woke up late, had a leisurely breakfast of everything your P.E. teacher told you not to eat, and hung around until check out time because I didn't have very far to go. That night, I would get to test out my tent for the first time on the trip.

I left the hotel and stepped into the muggy air. I was surprised how humid it was. It had rained the night before, and now the sun was drying everything up and the water on the road was evaporating to make steam that I was running through. It was very uncomfortable and immediately made me start sweating heavily.

My route wove in and out of tiny towns and then there was a gap between towns with some cattle fields and ranches. Before long, I reached the town I'd be staying in that night. As soon as I saw the sign welcoming me to Bryson, the sky darkened, the temperature dropped and it began to rain. I quickly covered my backpack with the rain cover and put on a jacket, but unfortunately, I wasn't able to do it fast enough without getting wet. I walked through the town looking for a restaurant to sit in so I could stay warm and dry until it got dark at which time I would go look for a place to camp. There was one restaurant in the town. I went up to it and the doors were locked. I looked at the hours and it was closed on Sunday and Monday. Which day was I there? Sunday.

I looked around at the worsening conditions and decided since it was closed on both Sunday and Monday, they probably wouldn't mind too much if I camped out behind their building. I called the first number on the door to ask and no one answered. I called the second number on the door and got a guy who didn't sound like he could understand me very well.

"Hello, I was wondering if I could set up my tent behind your restaurant just for one night."

"Huh? You want to park behind my building?"

"No, set up a tent. Can I set up a tent to sleep in?"

"An RV?"

"No, a TENT; like with poles."

"What about poles?"

I decided to change the direction of the conversation at that point.

"Thank you very much sir, I appreciate it."

"Umm . . . no problem!"

I wondered if I should sit there on the porch of the restaurant or just set up my tent quickly. I figured, it could only get worse, so I should set it up quickly. I looked around for any witnesses and bounded across the lawn to the back of the building just on the side of their shed. With fingers that were completely numb, and wet, I set up the tent as quickly as I could and threw my stuff in there. I sat there for a minute in my makeshift home and wondered what to do for the next 5 hours while it was still light outside. I changed clothes and put on my dry base layers that SmartWool had given me and got into my sleeping bag. For the rest of the evening I just read. I wanted to finish my book so that I could leave it somewhere and wouldn't have to carry it around anymore.

I couldn't help but feel a little bit like Bear Grylls chilling in my tent while freezing my butt off. The only difference was that when I looked outside of my tent I saw a lonely intersection in a town that was about 5 blocks long, and had most of it's "shops" evacuated and broken down. He had a view of Mt. Everest.

I went to sleep early that night after eating half of a loaf of peanut butter and jelly and several granola bars.

Chapter 49

Getting out of the sleeping bag while it was still freezing cold outside didn't exactly pose itself as an attractive option when I woke up the next morning. I was so cozy. I had my warm, dry SmartWool base layers on and was in a toasty sleeping bag. I ate some peanut butter and jelly's while still bundled in the bag and then I got dressed all while never leaving the warmth of my cocoon. When it finally came time to emerge, I got out quickly, packed up quickly, and took down my still soaking tent with my now numb fingers. I tried to start running as soon as I could to generate some heat, and before long, I was running comfortably at a decent clip.

It was still overcast and the temperature was very low. I don't know exactly what it was but if I had to guess I'd say it was somewhere in the high teens or low 20s with an annoying wind.

After rolling on hills for a good part of the day, I ran straight into two bikers with loaded bikes. Their names were Paul and Clint. Clint looked much younger than Paul, with good reason: he was. Clint was a blonde haired, blue eyed, thin, young guy who had just graduated high school. He squinted and sniffed a lot since it was so cold. His friend, Paul, seemed a little more comfortable in the cold. He had dark hair with a bit of gray peppered in, a graying beard, and wasn't quite as thin as Paul. They were biking from Maine to California to raise money for breast cancer. They called themselves "Team Bowditch."

We talked for a little bit about our routes, and how things were going, but we were all so cold, we didn't really want to stand around and talk while there was moving to be done. So, we parted ways and continued on our paths.

I ended the run that day in a little community called Runaway Bay where there was a body of water. It was the largest body of water I had seen since I left Huntington Beach. I was met by a man named Sam who would take me to his home to stay with him and his wife, Trish. They lived quite a ways away. He really drove out of his way to pick me up and drive me to his house. It was so cold; I really appreciated him doing that for me. Sam was a man that reminded me of Santa Clause; rosy cheeks and all. The only difference was that he had short hair, not long and curly. It was no surprise when I found out that he played Santa alongside his wife, Mrs. Clause at Christmas gatherings.

After arriving at their house, I took a hot shower that allowed me to thoroughly thaw out. I enjoyed talking to them about their grandson who has JRA. They told me his whole story. They were also very involved in the local Arthritis Foundation chapter and spent a lot of their time volunteering. Since we were very close to Dallas, the head of the Arthritis Foundation for Dallas came to their house for dinner and I was glad I got to meet Martha, who had donated a room a couple of towns back.

Dinner was delicious and Trish made sweet tea that was extra sweet. I was starting to really get used to sweet tea, and taking quite a liking to it. We had lasagna, salad, sweet tea, and cake for dessert. It was quite a difference from what I had eaten the previous night for dinner, and I went to sleep that night in a warm bed and a full stomach.

The next morning was just as cold as the previous morning. It even snowed a little bit. Trish drove me far out to where I had stopped the previous day. I can't say that leaving the heated interior of the car was as appealing as staying inside.

After thanking Trish and unloading my rig, I started off down the road into a bitter cold wind. I crossed the narrow bridge that goes over a very thin part of the lake and tried to get into a rhythm so that I could warm up some. Unfortunately, it was far too cold for that, and the majority of my day would be spent trying to run faster in hopes of a warmer body.

CHAPTER 50

That day I ran in some much denser populated areas. There were bridges that I crossed under that carried cars on highways. I ran through construction zones and along concrete barriers that completely erased any hope of a shoulder to run on. The cars flew on these roads and didn't seem to notice me or take any sort of precaution against coming within inches of my jogger and me.

It was an unnerving experience, and made me hate running on roads. Some cars honked as if I had a choice of being in their lane. Some cars paid no mind it seemed and even sped up to scare me. Well, it worked. While running over some of the overpasses I noticed a large amount of nails on the road and hoped that my stroller didn't get a flat because this would be the worst possible place to get a flat.

I saw the first neighborhood that had more than 10 houses in it since Phoenix and it looked like they were all the same house—cookie cutter houses. It reminded me of the east coast and how densely populated the space is. Just 50 or so miles back there was a town with space, so why did EVERYONE move right here? And why do they have to drive so fast. I started to feel myself questioning people's motives for living a fast paced lifestyle, always rushing around and honking at runners on the side of the road pushing a baby jogger. Why be stressed when just a couple counties away you could live on a ranch with space to breath, relax, and just be. Whenever I felt my mind start to wander and attempt to answer these questions I told myself to snap out of it, and pay attention to the *crazies* all around me.

In between densely populated areas, the country took shape again, yet the amount of people never wavered. It was during one of these sections where I saw longhorns, and it reminded me that I was still in Texas. As I neared the end of my day, I talked to the guy I was staying with that night and came up with a place to meet.

Before long, I met Michael of Denton, TX. He was an athletically built guy in his mid—30s, with a shaved head and a goatee. We loaded my stuff up and went on down the road toward his house. I didn't know much about him before I met him, only that he was a member of the local running club around Dallas. I learned that not only was he a marathon runner, he was a member of the 50 States Club; a club that someone can only join if they have or are in the process of running a marathon in all 50 states. I have met several people that were a part of this club, but most of them had only completed a couple of them. Not Michael. He was close to finishing. While I was with him, he was on number 35, and since then has completed several more, so he is very far along in his quest and will be accomplishing that soon enough. He is also an Ironman, which means he has completed the Ironman Triathlon. The Ironman Triathlon is a race made up of a 2.4 mile swim, a 112 mile bike ride, and a 26.2 mile run (a standard marathon). He had competed in several, and continues to compete in them throughout the year. On top of all his athletic achievements, he was a genuinely nice guy.

When we got to his house, he gave me the grand tour of his bachelor pad. The highlight of the tour was his TV collection. He and his roommate were sports fanatics and it clearly showed because they could never solve the problem of "which game to watch." They simply made a wall of 7 TVs, much like something you'd see in an electronics store, and tuned each one of them into a different game. He said that they used to have 9 but one broke, and one was just a loaner from a friend. It was very entertaining to see several games and the Olympics at the same time. Being the athlete he was, he got on his stationary bike for a while. I showered and relaxed before we met up with his friends for dinner.

We went to a Mexican restaurant for dinner that night and we had about 10 people at our table; many of them Ironmen. We had a good time eating large quantities of really good Mexican food. At dinner we made plans to meet up with Michael's friend Mike the following day so he could run with me for the first 14 miles of the day, at which point he would have to stop and go to work. I was happy to have someone along and looked forward to the next day's run. Not only would I have company, but it was also the last day until a 4 day vacation in Dallas, Texas with my dad's brother, Uncle Pete and my Aunt Nancy.

When Michael and I got back to his place, we made plans with his friend Chris for breakfast the next morning. I didn't know anything about his friend, but apparently, he was a big time runner.

CHAPTER 51

The Local Diner was a cool little place. When we walked in, I noticed a bunch of signatures on the walls and pictures of famous people who had eaten there. Musicians, actors, actresses, athletes, if they were famous, they signed the wall. Michael looked around the diner and waved at a man sitting at a table facing the window on the left side of the restaurant. Chris Phelan, at first glance looks like a mixture of a sea captain with his white hair and equally white beard, and an intellect. He had a certain air about him that gave me the impression he was very intelligent but was modest about it. His wire glasses rested on his thin face that gave away that he was some kind of endurance athlete himself.

Later on, I learned that back in his hey-day, he was the 8th fastest marathoner in the U.S. He is now a writer for the Phast Times, a magazine geared for runners, and triathlon enthusiasts and gives information on local athletes and races as well as interviews with various people Chris feels like writing about. I happened to be one of those people, so he asked to do an interview.

Pancakes are not something that I'm usually partial to eating right before I go for a 30+ mile run, but the ones Chris was eating looked so appetizing I couldn't resist ordering the same thing. While Michael and I chomped on our blueberry pancakes, Chris asked me various questions about the run, the reason, and how I was holding up physically, and mentally. It was different being interviewed by a fellow runner because he asked questions about certain running related ailments that a standard reporter wouldn't think to ask about. Fortunately for me, I hadn't been afflicted as of yet with any major problems, and I think this piqued his interest.

We sat and talked not only about my running but also what he does around the Dallas area in terms of running and biking. He started the Ride of Silence in

2003 after his friend, Larry Schwartz, was killed by a motorist while riding his bike. The idea behind the Ride of Silence is for everyone to ride their bicycles together at no faster than 12 miles per hour for at least 8 miles and not says a word in remembrance of those cyclists that have died while biking because of motorists. Since the first ride in Dallas, it has grown to include 317 separate locations and many different countries. As he explained how quickly the event had grown, I was in awe of the sheer numbers that came out to this event. There were no registration fees, no sponsors, and no talking.

He told me how powerful the past years had been, and how he was trying to get it spread throughout every state. There is even a ride in Antarctica! . . . on stationary bikes for those who were wondering how that worked. Chris was very interesting to talk to and I soon found myself asking him as many questions as he was asking me. When the time came to leave, Chris told the manager on duty what I was doing. The guy seemed like he lost his mind and said, "Dude! That's insane! You HAVE to sign our wall!" With a request like that, how could I pass up an opportunity to do something my mom taught me was wrong when I was two? I signed my name on the wall just to the right of the front door.

Chris rode with Michael and me to the spot 14 miles away from where Mike and I would start so we could leave Mike's car there. Mike got in the car with Chris, Michael and me to ride out to where we would start today's run. It was also nice to leave Mike's car there so that I could leave my jogger and not have to push it for 14 miles. If I didn't have to push it, why would I?

The air was bitter cold that morning, and the wind whipped our faces and our bare legs as we started running. Michael and Chris drove ahead a bit to take some pictures. After a few short stops I thanked them both for everything they had done for me and we parted ways for good. Mike was a jack of all trades. With the build of an endurance athlete, he had run marathons, ultra marathons, triathlons, Ironman, and long distance bike rides. Last year, he even had a friend run Badwater, and he went out for the race to crew for him. During ultra marathons, you are allowed to have a crew come to different aid stations to give you assistance with anything from changing your socks, to giving you special food, to helping to monitor your nutrition along with giving you a little boost of confidence when you feel like death has warmed over. Anything except give you a piggy-back ride to the finish. At Badwater, your crew is your life line. There aren't water stops every couple of miles, so without your crew, survival is not very likely.

I had tons of questions for him about the event, what it's really like there, and questions along those lines. Before I knew it, we were back to his car. Time always moves so much quicker when I'm running with someone. I took all of my supplies out of his car and once again, assembled my rig. I was getting good at putting it together pretty quickly at this point. We said our goodbyes, and I thanked him for coming out to run with me on a day with slightly less than ideal weather conditions; it still hadn't warmed up at all from that morning.

I started off down the road toward another group of people that I would run with before too long.

CHAPTER 52

In all the emails that my dad and I sent back and forth figuring out where I was staying, who I was meeting and where, and if someone was going to be running with me at all, the next group became known as "The Vicky's." No offense to Angie, but how many times do you come across two women named Vicky who are friends, and runners, and members of the same running club? Hence, "The Vicky's." The first Vicky spelled her name Vicki and she not only came out to run the last 5 miles of that day with me but also donated a hotel room a couple of days back. She was our point of contact with the people who were interested in running with me from the Dallas Running Club. She was able to round up two other women, Vicky, and Angie, to come out and put in a couple miles with me at the end of the day.

I kept running, and finally met up with Vicki, Vicky and Angie. They were a fun group, all of them full of energy and quite talkative, though not in the bad sense. All of them were avid runners and took part in many of the local races of all distances from the 5 kilometer race, to the marathon, that were put on by the Dallas Running Club. Angie, most notably, ran a marathon EVERY WEEKEND. She did so with no injury, and she loved it. When we talked about the races she had done, she always described the medal she received for finishing; especially the one she got for the Disney Marathon. She said it was huge!

Of course, before I realized it, we had reached the end of the 5 miles and it was time to say the goodbyes to the Vicky's and Angie, and meet up with my Aunt Nancy for a little vacation from the road. The last day of running before my little hiatus from the road went incredibly quickly. The first 14 miles with Mike had flown by as if we ran only one mile. The middle of the day, though chaotic from being in a very dense area with lots of traffic and no shoulder, went quickly because I was looking forward to running with the Vicky's. It also went quickly because I got so hungry I stopped at a Sonic Burger and filled my stomach to the brim with deliciousness. Eating large quantities of food while running was always entertaining, even if it was for no other reason than to see peoples' facial expressions.

CHAPTER 53

The next four days were spent with no running and much relaxing at my Uncle Pete and Aunt Nancy's house where I had a mini vacation. It was supposed to be my "body tune-up." A trip to the chiropractor to get an adjustment was spent trying to get the guy to stop laughing at me when I told him what I was doing. And a care package from my mom was at my uncle's house with more cookies and letters of encouragement. I felt a little bit like I was done because I did normal things while I was there. But in the back of my mind, I knew I had a long way to go, and it wouldn't be a walk in the park. The rest of the miles felt like a slight buzzing in my head kind of like you feel on the weekend when you know you have a lot of homework to do before class on Monday. It just nags you until you finish it. I read furiously in these days off. The book I was reading at the time was not particularly good, I just wanted to finish it so that I could mail it home and wouldn't have to carry it anymore.

After two days, I decided I couldn't take it, and went to the gym with my uncle. While a treadmill isn't quite like the running I had been used to in the past couple of months, it was good to get the motion down and feel like I was moving again, even though those miles didn't apply to the length of the country at all.

I thought that I had stayed pretty well in tune with what my body was doing. I hadn't lost much, if any, weight. I hadn't noticed my arms or shoulders decreasing in size. And my legs didn't seem like they'd grown any. I felt the same as when I started. On the road I had done a mild amount of push-ups and sit-ups to keep the muscles active and to try to prevent complete annihilation of upper body strength. When I was at the gym though, something didn't feel quite right. Lifting weights even half of what I was used to lifting on any given day before seemed very heavy now. I did the same exercises I had done before

I started the trip, but this time it seemed nearly impossible to complete the series of exercises I was used to doing. I was amazed at how weak I had gotten in just two months. I struggled the entire time we were there, and even began to feel a little bit dizzy; something I had never felt at the gym before. It was very strange, and a bit discouraging. This was the first big physical change I had seen since I started.

The weather was great the whole time I was there. It felt like fall: cool, sunny, slightly breezy, and the high of mid 60s in the afternoon. And it was dry—not humid like Virginia. Of course, on the fourth day, I checked out the weather and a cold front was coming through that would bring lots of rain. I didn't think much of it because weathermen had been wrong before.

CHAPTER 54

Waking up the next morning, I realized that the weathermen in Texas, as dry as it is, don't cry "rain" unless it's going to rain. So I got all of my stuff together that I would need for the day, including my rain gear. I would be leaving my jogger at the house because I was staying there again that night. My aunt drove me to the spot where I had ended 4 days earlier and I started running.

At first it wasn't all that cold and it wasn't raining all that hard. Unfortunately, that would change. I started off with just a jacket and shorts but packed my pants just in case. I didn't bring gloves because when I left the house that morning, it wasn't too cold and I thought they would just get wet anyway. Running down the soaked road, in and out of puddles, my feet quickly became water logged and I could feel the temperature drop significantly. I realized that I would need to add some covering for my legs and would also need to thaw out in order for my hands to work enough to put them on and retie my shoes. After about 15 minutes I found a Subway sandwich shop. I went in and asked for the bathroom still with my hat on and hood up because my hands didn't work well enough to pull off my hood. I was shaking pretty heavily and the guy looked kind of scared. I found the bathroom but needed both hands to turn the knob that in normal circumstances even a two year old could turn with little effort. I went in and immediately put my hands under cold water. I had to resist turning it to hot because my dad had warned me when I was little that the blood capillaries in your fingers can burst with too sudden of a temperature change. After a few minutes, I turned it gradually warmer until my hands were nice and toasty, and I had enough strength in them to put on my pants.

When I exited the bathroom, the guy behind the counter looked slightly less scared. He asked if I was okay, and I assured him I was by ordering a couple of cookies. I wanted to get as many calories in my system as I could before heading back out just in case my fingers stopped working again and I wouldn't be able to get eat any Gu's. The cookies were still warm. I could feel them enter my stomach still toasty and it felt like it warmed all my organs all at once. I thanked the man, pulled my hood back up, put on my CamelBak backpack, pulled my sleeves over my hands to protect them, and exited the safe haven. The wind hit me like a truck and the cold air rushed into the cracks between the skin of my face and the material of the hood and cold air circulated inside my jacket and instantly made me cold once again.

I started running as a lame attempt to stay as warm as I could. My feet were already soaked to the bone and before long would go completely numb. Little by little, more of my body became numb. First it was my feet and my face. The muscles in my mouth seemed to only know one shape: wide open. My eyes, though covered by sunglasses one of the few times I ever wore them, were so cold I tried to keep them closed with only minimal opening to try to protect them further. Then my calves went numb, then my knees, thighs, hips, and all of both arms. Pretty soon, I felt like a torso that was just moving down the road by leaning and hoping that, the extremities that were attached to said torso caught him before he fell face first on the wet asphalt.

On top of being very cold, I was stopped by the local police. I was running on the shoulder of a high traffic area in little or no visibility. I had my hood pulled up and tightened so that only my nose, mouth, and one eye were sticking out. I'm sure I looked like a creep but that's no reason to stop someone on the side of the road. He pulled up and signaled for me to stop. I stopped even though, moving was the only thing keeping me remotely warm.

He came up and very authoritatively yelled at me, "Remove your hood and show me some ID!" He said so in the same tone as I've heard officers in the movies say, "Put down the gun!"

"Yes sir, give me one minute, my hands are very cold."

"What the hell are you doing out here?" He said this like I was some kind of idiot who had cut in on his time in is warm, dry car. My excuses for fingers took forever to take off my pack, pull out my wallet and locate and remove my license. I explained I was running across the country.

The officer didn't even look up from reading my ID when I told him this like he didn't believe me. Why else would anyone with a Virginia driver's license willingly put himself in this kind of situation unless it was serving a bigger purpose?

He looked up after reading my ID like a novel and looked me straight in the eye and said very directly, "Do not. Go. Any. Where." He pronounced *anywhere* in two separate words and three separate syllables to show how serious he was. He walked slowly to his cruiser. I was getting colder by the second, and this guy was taking his time *checking me out*. When he returned he gave me my card back and asked what I was "actually" doing out there. I told him once again, and started to pull out one of the drenched business cards I carried around in the pack. I think he somewhat believed me but proceeded to ask me how many guns I was carrying. *Guns*, plural. I assured him I wasn't carrying any guns, yet he searched my tiny CamelBak anyway. Unsatisfied with the results of the search, he decided that as much as he wanted to bring me in for questioning about the *exact reason* for my being out there, he would have to let me go. I'm not sure why this guy wanted me to be a bad guy so badly, but it was difficult to deal with him.

I had several other "ride offers" the same day; four to be exact. One was an older couple who insisted I got into their car. I said, "Thank you very much, I really appreciate it, but I can't. I'm running to the Atlantic."

They pulled over and again insisted that they drive me somewhere.

"I am running across the country. I cannot get in your car. I do appreciate the offer though."

They just looked at each other and asked me again why they couldn't drive me. I explained why I was doing it, and why I couldn't take a ride, although it was very tempting; I could feel the heat from the heater coming out the window and slightly warmed part of my face. They still looked very confused and the guy said, "Alright" as he rolled his eyes and turned his head back toward the road in front of him.

The next guy slowed down his light blue pick-up truck and asked me if I wanted to get in his car. Again, I declined the ride, thanked him and kept on running. He kept driving slowly next to me, and I looked back toward his car and a very large man occupied the driver's seat. His left hand was guiding the steering wheel and on his left forearm perched a white miniature poodle. The little dog looked at me, and I looked at the dog, I looked back at the large man, and back at the dog. Some part of this scenario didn't quite play out quite right in my head. He asked me again, "Are you sure?" He dragged out all the vowels to make his offer seem even more appealing than it already *wasn't*. All I could think about was the scene in the movie *Silence of the Lambs*. I declined and remained focused on running forward. I was sure I didn't want a ride from anyone. And I was very sure I didn't want a ride from "poodle boy."

The last two people to offer asked quickly if I wanted a ride, and as soon as I declined bailed out. Something tells me if I had said yes, he would have still bailed.

On I ran, until I got to the intersection where I planned to meet with my aunt. I went into the only thing at the intersection, a gas station, and got a steaming cup of hot chocolate. I felt my blood start to warm, and I began to thaw.

CHAPTER 55

Back when I thought that I'd be doing mostly camping, and I wouldn't be interacting with people too much, I had a bit of a plan for the next section after I left my little vacation with my uncle. Katie was going to be on spring break soon, and said she wanted to come visit me while I was out on the road. I couldn't possibly turn the down opportunity to see her, so I planned to run as far as I could every day after I left my uncle's, so that I would be further east and she wouldn't have to drive as far . . . even though it would still be a hefty drive from Virginia.

As the run progressed, more and more people got involved and it was more vital to stick to the schedule. At first, this was slightly frustrating. Not frustrating because I didn't want to stay with or meet new people, but because sometimes I felt very good, and didn't really want to stop at 25 or even 35 miles. Days that were very nice became difficult to stop running at a predetermined distance.

Staying with people was also about strategy from a fundraising standpoint as well. People were more likely to mention me to their friends if I was staying with them than if they just read about me in the paper or saw my website. It would possibly come up in conversation, thus, driving people to the website resulting in possible donations as well as a possibility of another place to stay.

Because of the increased need to stick to the schedule, it was difficult to work my way around it so I could run further the week between my uncle and seeing Katie. When it came down to it, I was only able to add a couple of miles each day, thus not putting me much closer than a couple of miles to the east coast. This was a bit disappointing because a plan to help her out in terms of driving distance was a bit spoiled. I changed the plan to where I would run the predetermined miles each day. Then the day that I would meet her, I would run further while she was driving towards me, making one long day as an attempt to cut back on her driving by 15 or 20 miles.

CHAPTER 56

Following the cold rainy day turned out to be an interesting one due to injury, and figuring out how to cope with it. When I got out of bed that morning, my left knee didn't work. I could only bend it about 10% of normal when there wasn't any weight on it and couldn't put any weight on it if it were bent at all. It was quite painful. I hoped that it was just a soreness that would go away once my blood started churning, and things would flow a little easier. I decided not to tell anyone about it for fear that they would try to talk me out of progress that day, and any sort of doctor's diagnosis would certainly require me to take an actual hiatus from running; thus postponing and possibly preventing me from finishing.

Of course, this lack of mobility is not ideal for running . . . or walking for that matter. But I packed up all of my stuff and hoped for the best. I had a box to mail home and threw it awkwardly into the stroller and it wouldn't quite stay in. When I started the day it was cold and windy. I would've liked to run to try to stay warm but when I tried my leg literally wouldn't hold me up. It was ALMOST funny how it seemed that my leg would literally collapse under my weight if it were in any position besides straight and locked. I kept walking for awhile and my frustration kept growing. Every couple minutes I tried to run again and still, I would be forced to stop. I looked for a post office on my phone and found one in a couple of miles in a nearby town. I decided since, even on a knee that worked, running while holding a box on top of a stroller is awkward; so I would walk until I reached the post office and then would give running another go. I really hoped that by that point, my blood would circulate and would warm things up and everything would be okay. Then I would remember how cold it was and that the best way to warm up was to run; thus, establishing a wicked catch 22 that brought my spirits into a new low.

After reaching the post office and getting the box out of my hands I gave running another chance; again, no dice. Normally, I can run through these little problems. That day, it wasn't my choice. I would hobble for a minute or two and walk. Hobble for another minute or two, and walk. As the day went on and the blood was flowing a little more, things got a little looser. Pain subsided and I was able to tolerate more and more running mixed with walking. By the end of the day I had about 90% mobility and was able to run without stopping every 5 feet.

The day was supposed to be a 30 mile day but I decided to cut the day short by 10 miles and only do 20 miles in a last ditch effort to prevent further damage. I figured tomorrow I would make up the difference.

I think the knee issue was a result of my feet and legs being numb in the cold rain the day before and my stride going down the drain. I believe I ran on it wrong for 30 miles, and overnight it just fell apart as a result.

I found a tiny motel that was on the outside of town and got a room so I could shower, get out of the cold, and properly rest my aching leg. Luckily for me, I was there on a Tuesday and every Tuesday they had all-you-can-eat pizza at the local Pizza Hut for $5. I probably should have called ahead but I just showed up and so did the rest of the town. There were insane amounts of people in there and they were eating pizza just as fast as I was. There wasn't a whole lot of pizza on the buffet because as soon as they would put something up there would be a giant flock of people. Elbows would fly, kids were screaming, and by the time the dust settled, the pizza was gone. Perhaps that is a bit of exaggeration, and maybe I was the one throwing elbows and screaming like a two year old. No one knew me there, and I was eating by myself; there is a good chance my manners were not present. After too many slices of pizza to count, I retired to the room, tied some ice to my leg, elevated it and went to sleep. I knew I would have to wake up early to get a good start on the next day because there was a chance I wouldn't be moving very well, and I now had to go 40 miles to stay on schedule.

CHAPTER 57

I woke up the next morning with my knee slightly achy and mostly uncomfortable. It was the kind of pain I knew would subside once the blood started pumping. I checked the weather and saw that it was going to be sunny and cool: perfect for running. I started out about one minute before the sun rose. I was able to run from the start with a slight limp, but still, I was running. Running east all the time means that in the early morning, you are always running into the sun. The sun rose in front of me and I enjoyed the colors until it became too bright to look at.

The first 20 miles were spent running, enjoying the weather, and just enjoying the day. Then, I met a friend. I had a history of run-ins with dogs on the trip. And that day was no different except the run-in turned into a run-with. I was just humming along and then I heard this tapping behind me. I look down and I see this little white dog with a black head, and somewhat lighter brown ears running along side of me. I had to guess that he was some kind of terrier mutt. I told him to go home and that he couldn't come with me but I didn't see where he came from. He wasn't wearing a collar or tags or anything. When I stopped to tell him to go home again he just sat down, looked at me and wagged his tail. I thought if I just ignored him he would go away. I started running again and he stayed right with me matching my stride almost exactly. Every now and then he started to fall behind and then he would run a little faster to catch up with his bouncing ears and resume my pace.

I started to get a little nervous thinking I might need to find a place for him to sleep because he was staying with me. I decided since he wouldn't leave me, I'd name him for the day, or the rest of the trip if that's how long he stayed with me. I named him Paul, after Paul Bunyan. The way I saw it, Paul had an Ox and I had a dog. I'm not completely sure it made sense, but that's just what I named him.

Paul followed me for 20 miles. The dog could run. He would stop and sniff something and then come running back to me full speed. At one point he ran through a field that was next to the road I ran on. He chased other animals, and had a good old time. But whenever he was done investigating, he bolted back to me. Paul's one issue was traffic. For the most part he stayed right next to my left side but if a big truck passed he would hide under the moving jogger, making it a bit more difficult for me not to step on him or run him over. Every time this happened, I would stop and pet him, calm him down until his tail resumed its metronome-like steadiness and then we would continue on.

When we got to Paris I started to think of ways I could sneak him into the hotel so I could give him a bath. I had the plan all worked out. It would be great! I would leave the jogger downstairs just outside and I'd tie him to it. Then I'd check into the hotel, bring my back pack in and dump everything out in the room. Then I would go back downstairs and if he was still there, I'd put him in the backpack and bring him up to the room. I hadn't heard him bark yet, so I wasn't worried about him making noise. I had to figure out a way that I could keep Paul. If he could tackle 20 miles on a whim like this, I was sure he'd be fine for the rest of the country. It would be just me and my running dog, Paul; taking on the country. Well, we got to Paris, Texas and you know what they say, "Paris is the city of love." Paul agreed because he found himself a girl dog and ditched me. I guess he forgot who shared his water, granola bar, and crust from a PB&J with him. So, it was back to just me and the road again . . . and the stupid baby jogger.

The chamber of commerce in Paris, TX had helped me get a newspaper interview and so I met the interviewer at the local coffee shop before going to the hotel that was donated by a friend's parents. Afterward, I met up with Mindy who was the president of the chamber of commerce for Paris, Texas. She gave me a tour of the town and then we met up with her friend, Courtney for dinner. After dinner, Mindy showed me some more of the town and also showed me what they are famous for: The Eiffel Tower . . . with a cowboy hat on top. It was literally the Eiffel Tower, though slightly smaller, and on top of it, there was a giant red cowboy hat. Spotlights illuminated the tower at night, and Mindy told me it was a popular place for people to get married around there.

Another highlight from the day was I got two blisters. It was very weird, since I hadn't gotten any the entire trip yet. After I got back to the hotel, I addressed the issue and popped them. After I lubed the area well with antibacterial cream and wrapped them, they felt much better.

CHAPTER 58

I got a call early the next morning from Mindy to see if I was available to talk with the Paris high school. Of course, I agreed, and so she picked me up and took me to the school. They put me in the auditorium which I had never used as a venue before but as I got going, it was just the same old talking schpiel. They were all really nice, except they asked a lot of questions about hygiene. I thought I was clean but their volume of questions about showering made me think otherwise. Again, talking with the high school students was just like talking with my friends, just nice and relaxing. Afterward, I took off for my 30 mile day.

I ended in Clarksville and met Diane. She is the president of the chamber of commerce and had an incredible amount of energy. When I met her she had a very large Gatorade for me. The town of Clarksville wasn't exactly huge, so she took me on a walking tour of the town and hit all the major buildings in 3 blocks.

Her husband used to be the judge, so she was able to show me the courthouse which had recently been restored to its historical state and looked like something out of a movie. The courthouse also had a double set of stairs that led from the entrance to the main courtroom that was "technically" closed, but Diane didn't seem to mind the red ropes blocking our way. She hopped right over them, and I followed suit. When we entered the courtroom, it looked like I was stepping into an old movie scene. The bench and all the chairs in the whole room were completely wood. It was beautiful. There were huge windows lining the side of the courtroom giving the whole room just as much light as being outside would. Then she took me across the parking lot to the Courthouse Inn, where I would stay that night.

The Courthouse Inn didn't feel like a normal house. It looked like a cream colored dollhouse with red trim and a huge wrap around porch. I don't know much about styles of homes and what they are called, but if you can picture a doll house, you can picture the Courthouse Inn. Each room was themed just a little bit differently, but everything in the house was crafted beautifully. Most of the furniture was antique, but didn't give me the feeling that it would break if I sat in it. The house itself was very large with 6 bedrooms, a giant kitchen, dining room, foyer and two other rooms for sitting and talking. The house looked so nice; I didn't want to mess anything up. I felt bad bringing the stroller into the house, but I didn't know what else to do with it and the owner, Cheryl, instructed me to do so. She was a very nice lady and donated the room for the night. I didn't realize it at the time, but she didn't live there, and I was the only guest that night. This meant I had the whole house to myself.

While I was there with Cheryl and Diane, a reporter from the local newspaper came by and did a quick interview. Then, Diane showed me the Italian Bistro restaurant that I would be attending later that evening for dinner. The chamber of commerce donated the meal that night. After thanking Diane for setting everything up and giving me the grand tour of Clarksville, we parted ways and I went back to my room where I decided I was in dire need of a shower before I went to fill my belly with scrumptious Italian food.

When I walked into the bathroom I was greeted by a whirlpool bathtub! I was in awe of this house. While, at the current moment, I was feeling fine, and was more hungry than sore, I opted for the shower, but it was good to know the option was there. I then hiked the 3 blocks to the Italian Bistro and dined on some world-class chicken alfredo, garlic bread and a salad, all topped off with a now common order for me of sweet tea. I think I started drooling just ordering it. With how hungry I was, the order took forever, but in reality was very speedy. I took the first bite and immediately was transported to another dimension of tastes. It was a flavor explosion.

With a satisfied appetite, I walked around the town checking things out for myself in the comfortably cool evening. The town was quaint. It was the kind of place where everyone seemed to know everyone, but it wasn't a black hole of a town where no one came in and no one left. They had a main square where I was told they held festivals and it was surrounded by shops, many of which were under construction for renovations. I liked the town and everyone I had met was very kind.

CHAPTER 59

I was only down to 2 days before I would meet Katie. I had quite a few miles before the town of Magnolia, AR where Katie would be. But I still had stops to make before then. When I got to New Boston, TX, my dad's friend from the Marine Corps, Bruce, was there to meet me. I had heard many stories from my dad over the years about his friend. My dad first met Bruce in 1980 while they were in Officer Candidate School for the Marine Corps. He grew up in Bothell, WA. As a young man, he decided to be a teetotaler and not drink. Although this was different than most of the flight students, Bruce had no problem with friends because he was always the designated driver.

All throughout their flight training he would buy pasture land back in Washington and lease it to farmers. My dad was curious about where he came up with the extra money to buy land. While at Maguire's Pub in Pensacola, FL, my Dad had just returned from the restroom when Bruce said to him, "Desi, why don't you just drop $20 in the toilet in the beginning of the night, because that's where it's going to end up anyway?" My dad then figured out where the money for the land came from.

Bruce also became a pilot, but instead of flying helicopters, like my dad, he flew the A6 Intruder, the all-weather attack jet.

Now, he was able to travel around due to his work with Delta Airlines, and he had some family somewhat close to where I was. So he met me the morning I was supposed to run to Texarkana and offered to carry my jogger. I took him up on the offer because although Texarkana wasn't very far away from New Boston, the roads were terrible, there was no shoulder. The closer I got to the city more traffic picked up. It probably wasn't even a good idea for me to be running where I was, but if I had the jogger with me; it would have made things exponentially more difficult.

After I reached the city, I checked into the hotel room that was donated by the Courtyard Marriot and showered. Bruce said he'd wait for me and take me to lunch. He headed out afterwards en route to his family. I had never met Bruce before. Not only did he tote my jogger from town to town but he waited for me and then took me out to lunch. I found this to be the kindness from near strangers that I was learning to be slightly more common in the world than I initially had thought.

Chapter 60

I rose earlier than normal the next morning so I could start just before dawn to maximize my time in getting to Magnolia. Starting with a headlamp on, I made my way through the ghost town that Texarkana turned into overnight. Quiet city streets slowly became busier as I went and Texarkana, Texas became Texarkana, Arkansas just as it was starting to get light. As I crossed the border into Arkansas I was happy to see the biggest state I crossed now behind me. The giant took me 23 days to cross, including my days off, and the Atlantic Ocean was now more of a reality than ever. But even closer than that was Katie. She was only going to be 57 miles away, and I was well on my way to seeing her that day. Before long, I received a text message letting me know that she had left the halfway point between Virginia and Arkansas, and I picked up the pace. I was running well, fast, and strong. The problem is I was so focused on getting there as fast as I could; I was running too fast for the distance and ended up crashing a bit. And by "a bit" I mean I crashed hard. I ran out of energy, and little aches and pains turned into bigger aches and pains. I needed to get there, but first, in order to give me some energy, I had to eat. So I stopped at a Sonic burger and grabbed some burgers for the road. The energy was up, but my legs just wouldn't move as fast as I wanted them to.

After I had gone about 49 miles I got a call from her and she informed me that she was almost in Magnolia. We decided that I would finish the last bit of today's run at some point in the next couple of days; but for now, she would find me on the side of the road and pick me up.

Seeing Katie was within a few minutes' reach. The road seemed to curve on and on as I ran faster hoping that my attempt to cover ground would result in seeing her even sooner. As I came around one last curve in the road it became straight, very straight and long, and uphill. It seemed to be about 2 miles long.

There was a stop light up ahead that looked like it sat at the pinnacle of the hill. I ran toward it without taking my eyes off of it; studying each car's headlights looking for her Honda Civic's lights. Several of them passed me and I started to hate that her car seemed to be world's most common one. Finally, I reached the top of the hill just in time to see one more Civic, except this one pulled off the side of the road. The door opened and I saw her get out and run to me. I don't see her run very often, but she ran.

We must have looked like a couple of nut cases there on the side of the road hugging, but I didn't care. She was here. We packed up my stuff, looked around at the spot just so I knew where I stopped, and then we went to Magnolia.

Lesson learned, no matter how stoked you are for the finish line, respect the distance. I finished the day with another 50 miles under my belt.

CHAPTER 61

We decided that since we were in a part of the country neither of us had ever been before we should see as much as we could because there would be a fairly large chance we wouldn't have a chance to come back. Magnolia is in the very bottom left side of Arkansas which means it's also close to Louisiana. We had heard that Shreveport was nice, so we went down there for two days.

It was a nice little town, much less crowded than the busy east coast towns that we were used to seeing. The Red River goes right through the city with makes for a good spot for a boardwalk. They had paddle boats docked at several spots along the river but we couldn't decide if they were operational or not. Something else that Shreveport had was an IHOP and a casino. If you go at the right time of night, each can be equally entertaining.

We didn't do anything wild or crazy. We just stuck to the standard tourist, sightseeing, and hanging out, though, there was a casino. El Dorado, they call it; home of penny slot machines and a surprising amount of people over the age 65 winning, or losing, large amounts of moolah. It was a place in the world that still had cigarette machines and where, on a Wednesday evening, the majority of the city's population seemed to reside.

We figured we should challenge lady luck and try to beat her. After losing eighteen dollars between the two of us, we decided maybe gambling wasn't for us. Katie had to drag me out of there kicking and screaming though. Plus, we chose what slots to play based on the cartoon characters on the outside of the machine. Needless to say, we didn't know what we were doing and El Dorado didn't exactly give an instructional seminar on how to get serious about slot machines. I'd rather just find out where you're supposed to bump the machine to make the wheels stop so you win.

It was very nice to have the feeling of normalcy again. Being with Katie those couple of days gave me the feeling of being home, and it was good to be there. Unfortunately, the days passed quickly, and before I knew it, it was time for her to leave for Virginia. I was not ready to see her go, and wished she wouldn't. The end seemed so far away, and when she left, I wanted to go with her. It was the closest I ever came to quitting the run and just going home.

The day she left, I went back out to finish the last 7 miles to Magnolia. I ran out and back for a total of 14 miles, 7 of those being extra, and every one of those miles hurt. It was awful. When I finally returned to the hotel room, I just went to sleep. I couldn't wait to start running again so I could just get on with the end of this thing. There was still so much of the country to cover, and here I was sitting around.

CHAPTER 62

When I finally started to run again I ran from Magnolia to El Dorado which, I learned, was pronounced with a long "a." When I saw it written, I assumed it was pronounced the same way the "lost city of gold, El Dorado," was pronounced. A gas station attendant quickly set me straight after promptly stating that I wasn't from around those parts. I agreed and she told me how it was pronounced. El Dorado reminded me a lot of Old Town Fredericksburg, a town close to where I am from. Antique shops, bakeries, little old time drug stores, and a Christmas store made me think I had stepped out of the *Deep South* for a while. A red telephone booth, like the kind you see pictures of from England sat on one of the street corners. And there were little parks that took up about the same space as two stores. I made it a habit to walk through the towns so I didn't miss anything, and this was one town that I was happy to walk through. Even the people walking on the sidewalk smiled at me, though I couldn't tell if that's because they were expecting a baby in the jogger I was pushing.

I stayed at Union Square Guest Quarters Inn that evening. My room was more like a full sized apartment than a hotel room. The owner of the Inn donated the room when she heard I was coming through, and it couldn't have been any nicer. There were two large windows in the main room. One looked out on the main street, and the other was a patio that overlooked the courtyard. When looking at it from my patio, the side to the left of me was the street, the side to the right was an old train car-turned-restaurant where they served breakfast in the morning. Little white Christmas lights were hung around the whole square and it was quite pretty.

El Dorado was also the town where I met Dennis and Katherine, and their daughters, Amanda and Rebecca, as well as Tracy, one of the heads of the

Arthritis Foundation for Arkansas. Amanda has juvenile arthritis, and Dennis is a doctor. It was really interesting to hear their story because it was the first time I heard it from a doctor's point of view. The strange thing was it didn't sound much different from any of the other kids' stories I'd heard so far. I thought that since he was a doctor, it would've been a better scenario and they would have caught it sooner, known what it was from the start, and found a medicine that would help her right away. But, unfortunately, that wasn't the case, and it really showed me how strange the disease was, how sneaky it can be, and how not even a doctor for a parent would suggest arthritis in a kid at first symptom.

That evening we all went to a local Mexican restaurant and enjoyed some of the fine local eats. Katherine told me about her parents, who live in Louisville, Mississippi, who would later play a major role in my experience of Louisville (pronounce Loosvull). Having all the kids at dinner was fun. The normal kid catastrophes played a huge part in this. The problem of who had the color crayon the other kid wanted, who lost the game of tic-tac-toe, the spilled ketchup, and then the problem of the kids not eating enough. It reminded me of when my family was a little younger, and the scene looked quite similar.

After dinner we went back outside and the kids started running around like they had been cooped up for awhile. They had a long drive ahead of them, and they needed to get some energy out. One of them tagged me, so I had to be "it" until I tagged them. After a little while, they were good and worn out and ready for the long drive home. I would see Dennis and Katherine in a couple weeks at her parents' place in Mississippi, and Tracy was staying in the same inn as I was so I would see her and her son at breakfast the next morning.

CHAPTER 63

The train car the next morning had a very nice breakfast inside of it. Anything you could possibly want as a part of a continental breakfast was there. I opted for the granola and yogurt, fruit, a bowl of cereal with milk, a bagel, and a hardboiled egg. Even at breakfast I liked to put away large quantities of food. Tracy was heading back up to Little Rock and so we said our goodbyes, I thanked her for coming, and I went back upstairs to pack up.

I was in no hurry to check out because that night I would be camping. On days I was camping I wanted to reach the town somewhat close to dark so that if it was needed, I could set up my tent without being seen by anyone. When checkout time came, I went downstairs and met the owner who had donated the room to me. I was glad I got to meet her as she wasn't there yesterday to thank her personally. She asked me where I was headed and I asked if she knew anyone there. After a minute of hard thinking, she said, "Hmm, that's a very small town, but I believe I do know the folks who own Medlin's Hardware."

" . . . Is that right . . ." I inquired.

"Yeah, let me give them a call. They have a large field next to their store that they might let you camp in."

"Wow, thank you very much."

I'm not sure who she spoke to because later on that day when I went in and introduced myself, they looked at me like I was a crazy person.

Chapter 64

Before I made my way out of town, I wanted to see what else this little town had. I was lucky I did that because nearly two hours after breakfast, I was getting hungry again. Walking down the street, I saw a sign that said Elm Street Bakery. I simply could not resist. The aromas wafting through my nostrils called my name. Before I knew it, I was inside perusing the freshly baked goods. Fresh French breads, cookies of every size, color and flavor, croissants, cakes, and pies stocked the bakery's shelves. It was a smorgasbord of deliciousness, and my eyes wanted to try everything. My stomach knew it was a bad idea right before running, even if it was only 20 miles. After walking around the shop for several minutes deciding what would be best, weighing my options, and compiling mental pros and cons lists for each possible item. I came up with no cons to anything except the sheer amount of sugar in each delectable choice. I decided to go with something that I hadn't had before but I knew would be insanely scrumptious. The strawberry and cream cheese filled croissant. I knew that my palate would thank me for this decision even if my stomach did not. Besides, I decided that the choice would taste somewhat reasonable if it made a second appearance later on in the day.

I ordered it, and I saw the girl slide the glass door open. There was now nothing blocking me from jumping over the counter and devouring the entire tray of them. She grasped the tongs in her hand and placed the ends around the pastry that would soon be mine. When she squeezed the flaky crust of the croissant I could see each end slightly compress and some of the flakes overlap. I prayed that every flake stayed on so that I could thoroughly enjoy every calorie that would enter my mouth. She placed it delicately on a small plate and handed the monstrosity to me. As possession of the baked good transferred from the girl behind the counter to me I felt the weight transferred to me as well. Surely, the plate wasn't this heavy. There must be more filling than I thought. It was finally in my hands. My mouth began to water. I could almost taste it. I walked casually over to the cash register to pay for it making sure my steps were not too quick as to rush the girl behind the counter. I didn't want her to know how much I was anticipating what I was about to enjoy. She didn't say anything to me, just pressed buttons on the machine. Finally after what seemed like an eternity, she opened her mouth to say, "That'll be $2.48."

"$2.48 .... $2.48 .... " I said it over and over again in my head. How could I be so stupid as to not have $3 waiting to give to her while she plugged the price into her magic money holding box?? Trying to move calmly to not seem anxious, I set the plate holding my soon-to-be enjoyment down on the counter to take off the CamelBak backpack that I held my wallet in. I scrambled to get the money from my brown, Italian leather wallet.

"How could you be so stupid? Why didn't you have the money ready? Okay, calm yourself. It's just a croissant . . . Yea, but it's an awesome croissant! Wait, am I answering myself in my head? Why, yes you are, Patrick." Arguing with myself in my head was starting to creep me out.

I handed the girl behind the counter the money and she gave me my $0.52 change. As I turned toward the door to find a seat and chow down I heard a voice behind me ask, "Did you want a fork?"

A fork? Do I want a fork? For a croissant? Not normally, but this way I can politely shovel every atom of that thing into my mouth. After debating with myself, I decided I did indeed want a fork and so I replied, "Yes, thank you, I would."

Now I was all ready to enjoy my treat. Several empty seats called my name but I chose one near the window where I could people watch and keep an eye on the jogger. I sat down with fork in hand. There was nothing stopping me from trying to shove the entire thing in my mouth in one bite and only using the fork as a tool for prying my mouth open wider to thoroughly get it all in there. Or I could use it the same way you would use a shoe horn, just to lay it on the inside of my cheek and shove with the other hand. I was about to be polite and remember my manners when a little piece of color caught my eye. It was on my stroller, and my peripherals didn't recognize it. I paused, looked up, and saw that it was just the paperback book I was reading. I had read much of it this morning in a desperate attempt to finish it before I left the hotel room so I could just leave it there. I was very close to finishing it, and could probably finish it right now.

182

I glanced back down at the untouched heaven-filled pastry. Do I dare get up, get my book as a sort of masochistic torture devise to deprive myself of the one thing that I had been craving so hard for at least the past 2 minutes and 4 seconds? Yes, I dare.

I got up and left my croissant on the table, went outside to fetch my book, returned to the table and opened the book to the page with the dog ear folded in the corner of it. The part of me that enjoys pain a little bit was laughing at the part of me that wanted to take the biggest bite of my life. I found the sentence I had last read, and simultaneously picked up my fork. Without looking, I turned the fork sideways in my left hand and pressed down on the corner of my recent purchase. Still without looking, I turned the fork over and stabbed the piece I had cut. Part of me was enjoying how torturous this all was. While reading a sentence out of the book, I placed the pastry skewered on the fork into my mouth.

Immediate disappointment. It was dry, and there was no filling. Though light, flaky, and deliciously buttery, it was not what I was expecting.

On the verge of tears out of sheer disappointment, I looked down at the pastry that at one point I held such high hopes for. On the plate, though, replacing the corner I had recently dismembered from the rest of the heap of pastry was an obscene amount of strawberry filling and cream cheese flowing. I had only released the beast that was within! With a newfound hope, I moved my fork to the other end to unleash that end of the mayhem of filling. Again it tasted light, flaky, and buttery, but no filling. And from the opposite end, a river of filling flowed. I felt like Jed from the Beverly Hillbillies striking black gold.

With the ends now gone, I had a nice ratio of filling to flaky going for me. I sliced off a small piece making sure to get the croissant, cream cheese, a good piece of strawberry and the strawberry sauce on my fork. With all ingredients together on my fork I eased the pointy metal transporter into my open palate. Closing my mouth and pulling the fork out, there was nothing between the combination of ingredients and my taste buds. Immediately the mixture began to flow throughout my mouth and all of my taste buds danced. The flavors were intoxicating, and soon, my sense of smell joined the party of senses affected by the medley of food. It was purely delectable. With every bite another sense joined the group until my ears even heard an orchestra playing some grand tune with every instrument harmoniously in tune with the group of flavors. It could have been the music playing in the bakery but I would rather think the strawberry and cream cheese filled croissant was just *that* good. I ate it slowly and in very small bites so that I could make it last as long as possible. After finishing the masterpiece of culinary genius, I exited the Elm Street Bakery in a slight daze trying to understand how anything in the solar system could taste that good. Since I finished my book, I asked some random person on the street if they had read it. They had not, so I gave it to them. While this might sound slightly odd, it was mainly for selfish reasons. I didn't want to carry it anymore.

CHAPTER 65

No matter how much you walk or run the distance, twenty miles just doesn't take that long to complete in terms of trying to burn sunlight. I was happy, however, to learn that I found Medlin's Hardware without any difficulty. I went inside to talk to someone about setting up camp in the field next to the store. I introduced myself and mentioned the owner of the inn that I had stayed in, and it didn't seem to be ringing any bells. So I started over. I introduced myself and told the man what I was doing. I asked him if it would be okay if I set up my tent in the field next to the hardware store. He said that would be fine and introduced himself as Mr. Medlin, the owner of the store. I thanked him and left to wander the town for awhile so that I wouldn't be as noticeable during full daylight.

I grabbed a bite to eat and while I was sitting outside at the picnic tables I had some great conversations with a few people. One of them was a park ranger who worked up the road about 20 miles. He was thinking about training for a marathon.

"I ran one on a whim, sort of like a dare last year."

"On a whim? That's awesome! How'd you like it?"

"I had such a terrible experience and it hurt so much. I never wanted to do it again. But lately I've been thinking I may give it another go, and this time, maybe I'll train for it."

Luckily, I was there to reassure him that actually training for one may enhance his experience a little bit. He said he would, and seemed stoked enough on it to actually follow through.

"By the way . . ." he said as he turned to leave, " . . . there was a guy who passed through the town a couple of days ago who was riding a big covered wagon that was being pulled by a horse. All I know about him is that he was from Texas and was traveling the country by horse and wagon, the way the settlers did . . . except with a nice paved road."

I thought it sounded pretty cool, and thought to myself, *I may catch up with this pioneer.*

As it started to get dark it got cooler and I was ready to set up camp and climb into a warm sleeping bag. I climbed into the down bag and felt the temperature drop around me as I quietly munched on a couple of peanut butter and jelly sandwiches and read by headlamp before I went to sleep.

I was laying there in my tent and I heard a car pull up in the field where my tent was. I start thinking to myself, *Please don't be the cops, please don't be the cops.* I heard a car door open and someone's feet hit the ground. A person walked around the vehicle and toward my tent. I couldn't see anything because I was inside my tent not wanting to unzip the door flap. A man's voice asked, "Is anyone in there?"

I quickly responded, "Yes, give me one minute."

I climbed out of the tent to see Mr. Medlin standing there.

He said, "We thought you might be hungry, so we brought you some dinner."

Walking over to the passenger side door, his wife rolled down the window and handed me a big plate of food. I was in shock. I talked to the couple for a little while and learned that Mrs. Medlin she said she saw me earlier in the day. At first, she thought I was homeless. But then she said my legs looked a little too fit to be a homeless person's legs.

They asked if I ever talked to schools, and if I would be interested in doing that the next day because she was a teacher at the local elementary school. Of course I was, and so we made plans for the morning. As if that wasn't cool enough, it was shake-n-bake chicken which is one of my favorites. Mrs. Medlin apologized because it wasn't fried chicken, but they are watching their cholesterol. After bringing me dinner, I couldn't believe she was apologizing for anything. There was also corn, salad, bread, and a little personal pie as well. They brought me a Mountain Dew, but I decided that should probably wait until morning due to the caffeine.

CHAPTER 66

The following morning, I woke up and packed up, and wheeled the jogger over to Medlin's Hardware so I didn't have to fold it up and put it into Mrs. Medlin's car. She picked me up and brought me out to Gardner-Strong Elementary. I entered the cafeteria where the whole school, it seemed, was already there. They looked at me with wide eyes as I, a slightly dirty and disheveled looking guy with very tan skin and shorter than average shorts, walked from the back of the room to the front where their principal welcomed me. She introduced me and I began my standard dialogue telling them about where I had started, where I would end, and why I was doing it. I basically just ran down the regular interviewer questions of who, what, when, where, and how, threw in a few stories, strange sights and facts, and then opened it up for questions.

I remembered that elementary school aged kids liked asking questions about where I went to the bathroom but thought that I should keep the potty-talk for during question time because if I threw it in the part where I was just telling them about the run, the teachers might get a little freaked out that the dirty strange guy was talking about using the bathroom to a group of little kids. I figured I would ease up on the creep status and save those stories for question and answer session.

This group seemed more focused on other things though. They asked questions like "What's the farthest I've ever run?" and "How much water do I drink?" My favorite question, though, was "How much can you bench press?" I had no idea. The little boy who asked the question looked like he weighed about 40 lbs so I just said, "Um . . . Two of you." I'm not sure if it was true or not but it could be. It seemed that every kid in the place had a question but I couldn't answer them all in the time they gave me, so after answering as many questions as I could I said goodbye and Mrs. Medlin drove me back to the hardware store where my gear was. I was incredibly thankful for all they had done for me; let me camp out on their property, fed me, and brought me to the school so I could talk to the kids of the town. I couldn't believe that all of this was done by a couple of people who had never heard of me, known I was coming, related to me, or even knew I existed until I walked into their store.

As soon as I started running that day, I thought hard about the trip so far. Except for a few minor aches and pains, I hadn't been seriously injured, I hadn't had any major run-ins, no one had hit me with their car, and everyone I came in contact with helped or wanted to help me in some way. Things were going smooth, and the end seemed closer than ever. I had the run that day, then one night of camping, then the town of Lake Village, a day off, and then I crossed the Mississippi. I was feeling very optimistic and was on a serious "finishing high." I had this in the bag, all I had to do was stick to my routine, relax, and have fun. No sweat.

Approaching Crossett, AR I noticed even more logging trucks than I had seen lately. As the amount of trees lining the road increased, it seemed the amount of logging trucks increased as well. Getting closer still to Crossett, a number of paper mills popped up, and reaching Crossett I noticed the smell of a paper mill. I didn't know that's what it was at the time, but the smell of sulfur was very prominent throughout the town because of the paper mill.

I ran through the town and found the donated hotel I was staying in that night. When I went to the front desk I checked in, and really wanted to question the stench of the town but didn't want to offend the place she called home. Upon finishing everything transaction-wise she said, "Enjoy your stay, and enjoy the smell!" I knew the question was fair game at that point, "Yea, what is it and why does it smell like sulfur?"

"Hunny, that's the paper mill. It's just beyond those trees over there." She pointed to a spot in the direction I had just come from.

"Oh, that makes sense, thank you."

I had never smelled a paper mill before, nor had I been to a paper mill town. Two things I could cross off my experiences list, whether I wanted them crossed off or not.

Very close to the hotel I was staying at was a Huddle House Restaurant. I decided to go there for dinner because the other choice was Mcdonald's. I walked in with my book in hand ready to feast on some brinner: breakfast for dinner. I snagged a seat and cracked my book again, hoping to gain some ground in it. I enjoy reading, but when you're trying to travel as light as possible, sometimes carrying books is not the way to do it. I sat there surrounded by people who were slightly older than me by about 70 years or so, and the waitress came up and took my order for a pile of pancakes. I love pancakes.

Sitting around a Huddle House alone, in running shorts, surrounded by people who look like they are old enough to describe how dirt was created, I guess I drew some attention to myself because the waitress asked me what I was doing in that town. I told her and she immediately launched into the summer she remembered *back when she was my age*. She talked about it like it was a thousand years ago but I did not think she was much older than mid 30s.

She went on a bit of a rebellious spree and "slightly" ran away from home. I wasn't sure what "slightly" meant but I took it for either, "I ran away from home, but told my parents I was doing so," "I ran away from home but was old enough to do so without it being a problem," or "I ran away from home but no one really cared too much." She told me how she hitch hiked across the country for several months just going around and seeing stuff. Her story sort of reminded me of the sequence in Forest Gump where Jenny was hitch hiking around, being a hippy, and trying some psychedelics, which after talking to her, wouldn't really surprise me much if that sequence was a narration of her time on the road. "Things were different back then. You didn't have all these 'crazies' blowing stuff up and stabbing people right and left. Hitch hiking was generally pretty safe, and I didn't have one bad experience the whole time on the road. But you, kid, I don't know how you're still alive."

I thought two things after talking to her. One: I haven't met "all the crazies out here" yet . . . I wonder what I'd do if I met a "crazy."

And the second: I haven't had a bad experience yet either . . . maybe things aren't as different as people say. Maybe our parents, who were raised in the 60s and did the hitch hiking and "crazy stuff," were the ones who made all the stories about the killers on the road. Maybe they made up how unsafe it is to travel that way so that their kids wouldn't do all the stuff they did. Maybe they didn't want us to make the same "mistakes" they did, and fear was the only way to get us out of trying to see the country without the safety of our own vehicle. Or maybe, people just aren't as bad as we make them out to be. I liked the last possibility.

Returning to my hotel room that night, I thought about what makes someone fear something enough not to do it. Is it the consequence? That clearly isn't the case for some of the people sitting in prison right now. Was it something like pain? Is that why more people didn't run across the country? I caught myself starting to question more things and I decided to put an end to it quickly. It's not that I didn't want to think about it then, I just wanted something to think about the next day. I wrote myself a note so I didn't forget what I was thinking about. I would have lots of time to think because I'd be alone all day, and I'd be camping tomorrow night on the side of the road. For some reason, I thought I'd need material to keep my mind busy, even though, I've never had trouble with that before.

CHAPTER 67

The next morning I woke up late, as I liked to do on days that I knew I was camping. I went into the hotel lobby because they said they had a continental breakfast and grabbed a handful of packaged muffins. Walking down the road I inhaled one of them without even looking at it. As I opened the second one, I looked at it, and it was covered in mold. The third one didn't have too much mold on it, and I was still hungry so I just scraped the mold off of that one and still ate it. The second was a lost cause. I did, however, wonder how much mold the first one had on it, and how much homemade penicillin was floating around in my system at that moment.

Without anything to look forward to that night, I settled into a very slow pace just trying to burn daylight. Thinking about the questions from the day before, I quickly linked them back to my task at hand. My thought process quickly became negative and focused inward on how much I missed familiarity, and my family. My mood plummeted.

Mood swings from day to day were about as common as the sun coming up every day. I never knew what thoughts would make me start thinking about the vastness of the land I still had to cover, and the uncertainty of completing it. I didn't understand why I would start to have highs and lows in rapid succession during a single day's run. In the later miles of an ultra marathon I've heard of people having huge mood swings that make them get so low they are barely moving to so high, they drop whoever they are running with. Personally, I had not experienced this in a race, but I was feeling it now. Just yesterday I was on top of the world. Everything was good and nothing could get me down. Today was not that day. I took off my watch so that I would stop looking at it, put my head down, looked at the white line passing underneath my joggers rear right tire, and I ran. The only thing I could hope for was a place to safely set up my tent and to get there at the same time it was getting dark.

There wasn't much between my starting and ending points but at about 3:30 I looked at my watch and came across a Mexican restaurant. I saw it from a ways back and planned on stopping to eat because I wasn't sure what was around my stopping point. Besides, I could really use the break. They had a huge banner outside proclaiming, "FAJITAS ONLY $5.99!!"

My first thought after reading that sign was, "Done deal."

I parked the stroller and went inside. It smelled like heaven: fried Mexican goodness just waiting to be devoured. There were two other customers in the whole restaurant. I didn't think anything of it since it was a strange time of day. The women sitting across from me spoke in hushed tones in their booth and leaned in toward each other when they were talking. They must have really not have wanted me to hear anything they were saying. It was slightly awkward but I didn't mind too much.

When the waiter came over he handed me a menu. The truth was I didn't need the menu, I already knew I was getting the fajitas but figured I could burn some more daylight scoping the items for awhile while I munched on the inhuman sized basket of warm chips and salsa. When the waiter came back I ordered the chicken fajitas. Just saying it made my mouth water.

I sat there and looked out the window at the road that was part of my route and thought about if anyone knew that this road is part of a route to the Pacific Ocean. I asked myself the question and forgot about answering it almost as quickly as it popped into my head. I didn't really care. I could hear the fajitas before I could see them. Sizzling behind the kitchen door, it swung open and the waiter came out with a steaming hot iron skillet, and several other plates. I liked the way this looked. He came out like he was carrying an order for 6 people all at once, and yet, it was all my order; AND I was getting it for $5.99. Bonus.

Soon after devouring the massive portion of food, I decided to resume running. As I made my way through the rest of the town, my mood fell even further. I didn't understand how it was possible. I had just eaten a delicious filling meal, and now I felt even worse mentally. I expected to maybe have a stomach ache, or feel like a slug, but mentally, I thought I'd be back to normal. Nope, not today.

The decision to keep moving wasn't really my own. If I had found a half decent hiding place right then, I would have set up camp and gone to sleep in hopes that it would help me to wake up in a better mood the next morning. But, there was no such luck. There was an alternating pattern to the scenery. First there would be a grouping of 10 or 15 houses. It would be followed by farm land with no trees anywhere in sight. Then a couple miles would go by and more houses would pop up, followed by more farm land. This was all happening on the flattest land I had seen in quite some time. I was starting to wonder where I would camp that night. Uncertainty dragged me further down. I tried to relate myself to the kids with arthritis who had "down days" all the time with no end in sight. At least I had some ending in sight, even if it was still several weeks away.

During one passing of a group of houses I saw a man walking from his car to his house looking like he was returning from work. He said, "Ya look like you've been running for awhile!"

I was thinking, "Yes! Hopefully you will invite me into your house and I will get to take a shower!" but settled for, "Yes sir, since the Pacific Ocean."

"Geeze! I was thinking like 10 miles!" I stopped to talk to him hoping that some light conversation would result in a place to stay. We talked about why I was doing it, how long I'd been out there and the likes but no such luck. After awhile, he said, "Well, the wife probably has something good for dinner tonight, I'd better be going. Where you staying anyway?"

"I have a tent, do you know of anywhere to camp up ahead?" Hoping the guy wasn't just teasing me with dinner comments.

"Eh, not really, it gets a bit more wooded up ahead but not really. Take care now, stay warm, it's gonna be cold tonight."

All I could muster was, "Thank you." That brightened my mood. It truly did. For some reason that guy didn't invite me to stay with him, and I decided it was because I didn't look as pitiful as I felt, and he had faith in me that I'd be okay. Either that or I looked so pitiful that I looked insane and the guy was thinking, "There's no way I'm letting this loon in my house." I stuck with the first.

After several long miles of this pattern I saw the group of trees up ahead where I saw the road go into and cars on the road disappeared. I hoped there weren't houses there and it would be some place for me to hide out because the sun was starting to set and I was in no mood to run at night. Entering the wooded area, I saw a gravel clearing with a hill on the left, looked around really quickly and jumped up it. The other side was slightly cleared, mostly flat and had a ton of trash all around it. I decided it would do. I ran back to my jogger, looked around again, and sprinted for the hill. Once I was on the other side I kicked away the trash and thought it was funny that there was an abandoned old toilet there. My mood was brightening and I found it comical that the only camping spot I had seen had a bathroom with it. I had no idea that I would think about using it later.

CHAPTER 68

As darkness fell over my makeshift campsite, I was happy I found it. I had privacy, I was safe, I was warm in the sleeping bag, and I was only mildly hungry. I decided that I would eat a peanut butter and jelly sandwich, do a little reading, and call it a night.

Since my sleep schedule was slowly getting stranger, I couldn't get to sleep that night. I laid there wide eyed and listened to the sounds of the woods and even though they were soothing to me, I couldn't sleep. I finally got tired around 11:30 when I looked at my watch for the last time. Not long after that, I fell asleep.

At 1:00 am I woke up very suddenly with a large ache in my stomach. It was the kind of stomachache I only get if I'm either really hungry or really sick. I had the loaf of peanut butter and jelly right next to my head so I started to open that but I didn't feel like eating. Then it hit me . . . *I'm going to barf.* I unzipped the bag as fast as I could, instantly breaking out in a sweat and getting chilled because the air outside the sleeping bag was frigid. As more and more saliva started gathering in my mouth I pulled on my shoes and tore open the first zipper of the tent, and pulled the zipper for the rain fly as hard as I could. At the same time I jumped up, grabbed my headlamp, slipped on the down-filled sleeping bag and fell out of the tent shirtless and only in running shorts onto the damp, cold leaves. I turned over just in time to crawl furiously on my hands and knees as far away from the tent I could, which turned out to be only 5 feet, before a geyser of fajita and stomach acid hurled from my open mouth.

Every muscle in my body seized and my head felt like it was splitting right down the middle. Wave after wave of burning liquid evacuated my body. After I was done I stood up on shaky legs and drenched in sweat. I opened my eyes as wide as I could and turned on my headlamp. Everything I saw was blurry. I stood up and my sight began to return. I looked at myself to see if I needed to clean anything off of me. Miraculously, I had done all of that without getting even splashed by the tsunami that was my puke. I was relieved and slightly worried at the same time. When I looked at my arms and legs I was able to see every vein in all four appendages as well as in my stomach and chest. It looked like I had been turned inside out. Slightly disgusted, with a swirling head, and still shaking knees, I got back in the tent and hurried to get into the sleeping bag to warm up.

Knowing that would not be the only occurrence tonight, I put on more clothes so that I would at least be clothed when round two came. Unfortunately, it came sooner than I thought. Within 5 minutes, I was diving for the second zipper again. After that time, I just left my headlamp on. Soon enough, it was the other end's turn and I was rummaging as fast as I could through my bag for toilet paper, just barely finding a tree to hold onto in time for the geyser to explode out the other end.

Every time I thought I was done, another wave would hit. In and out, in and out, in and out; barf, crap, barf, crap, barf, crap. The cycle never ended. In between barf sessions I would lay there in the dark, curled up, trying to reserve some heat so that I wouldn't become hypothermic from being soaking wet with sweat in the cold when my body's defenses were already down. I was a decrepit mess. *How was I supposed to run 23 miles to the next town in a few hours? I can't sleep, I have no calories in my system, I can't just drop my pants on the side of the road in someone's yard and just let things go, things can't get any worse.*

The funny thing is that whenever I think to myself, *things can't get any worse*, they tend to get worse. During one break from the barf and crap-fest, huddled in the sleeping bag, I heard a sound that I had heard only a couple times in my life, and never in quite this setting. It was the sound of a coyote howling. First, it was one, then it was many. It was hard to place a number on them because they were quite far away at the time. They were losing their minds over something, barking, yipping, and howling. And then they stopped. I wasn't too worried because they seemed far enough away not to pose a threat. About 10 minutes passed with complete silence other than the barfing noises I was making. Then they started again. First, it was one, and then they all chimed in; this time much closer. I guessed that there must have been any number between 10 and 25 of these things. I realize it's a pretty wide range for a guess but I thought if 10 of them tried really hard, they could sound bigger, or it was 25 of them not all howling at once. They continued barking, yipping and howling; and just like the first time, they stopped.

This time I was slightly more worried, but not to the point where I was actually scared yet. It just seemed weird and maybe they were hunting something, but I didn't expect them to come and mess with me. Another 10 minutes of silence passed, and I needed to evacuate the tent again. This time I tried my hardest to blow chunks with grace and be as quiet as I could. At this point, though, I was down to stomach acid, and having my body force that out was tough as is. Trying to do it quietly was out of the question. I was sure they would have heard me, known I was weak and taken it upon themselves to get a 155 lb meal out of me. As soon as I was done, I stood up on wobbly legs and felt dizzy. Once I regained some balance, I scampered back to the safety of my dome vinyl force-field and turned out the headlamp. Sitting there in the dark knowing that a pack of cunning predators was in the area made me feel a little like the people in the movie Jurassic Park just sitting there and waiting for the inevitable.

Not 30 seconds passed before I heard the one coyote start yipping soon followed by all the others; this time, even closer. I wasn't a very good judge at how far away they were the first time, and even worse judge at how close they were now, but I knew that now they were close enough to get scared over. I could feel my stomach churning, which meant another bout of the fury was going to need to be released from the chamber soon enough. I tried to keep it in, but finally realized there was no use in holding it, and it would need to escape. A final mad dash toward the outside resulted in a successful and clean bowel release. With the headlamp on, I pointed it in the direction I expected the marauders to be coming from if they were that close. I held completely still and could see my breath dance in front of the headlamp. I was petrified and yet was stuck out in the cold, still wet, with my pants around my ankles gripping with all the strength I had onto a skinny tree. Upon finishing my business once more, I returned to my pop up home and once again, waited.

One minute after I climbed back into the sleeping bag and resumed my fetal position for warmth I heard crackling leaves and breaking twigs echoing in the surrounding woods. I was sure they had surrounded my tent. The sound of snapping sticks got louder as they got closer. My make shift home was surrounded by regurgitated food. My dog at home would have been drawn to it; I thought for sure they would be too. I was able to guess they were within about 100 ft. I buried my head under the sleeping bag to muffle my breathing. I breathed delicately and so quietly, even I couldn't hear it. The group of hunters was on my left side moving in what seemed to be a line moving passed me. They were still within about 100 ft, but didn't seem to be getting closer. My stomach churned and gurgled loudly, signaling a need for relief soon. I decided to focus on not letting that happen for awhile, and prayed that decision was actually up to me.

Listening to them pass me by, I guessed there were about 5 or 10 now that they were close enough to hear them move through the woods. Then, completely unprovoked, they stopped. One let out a howl, and no more than half a second later the rest of them chimed in. The collective song of the predators was petrifying. No, not petrifying. There is no word for the sheer terror I felt. My heart stopped and I thought about the fact that this was how I would meet my Maker. The inside of my eyelids flashed visions of certain points in my life like they were projection screens and my brain was the projector. I was sure the dogs were signaling the pack to move in on me for the final kill, and it would have been an easy one.

Suddenly, a goose started squawking and making lots of other goose noises! The sound of squawks, yips, barks, and shuffling leaves flooded the dead sound of the woods at night. 4:30 am was no longer a quiet time. Growls and sticks breaking echoed, and then the goose let out a deafening noise that I had never heard. I could only imagine it had been caught. Several seconds of haunting sounds of a goose dying at the paw and jaw of a coyote drowned out the sound of my stomach gurgling. It didn't take the hungry hunters long to devour their latest meal. Listening to them yip and bark at each other over who got what only lasted for a couple of minutes. They had hunted, killed, and eaten in a very short time. I only hoped that they kept moving the direction they were moving in and didn't decide to add fajitas and guys named Patrick to their menu.

Lying there, I wondered what I would do if they jumped me. I wanted to go through an awesome sequence of me taking on multiple coyotes in an epic battle where I was able to strangle one, and use his body to block the rest of them. Then I'd find a sword amid all the trash and fight them off bravely only receiving scratches in aesthetically convenient places like on the top and bottom side of my eye, on one shoulder and one pectoral. They would make excellent scars that would give me instant brave warrior status that the ladies would faint over. In this sequence, I was also a muscle bound Viking-looking dude with a massive beard and long hair, and it all took place in slow motion.

In reality, though, I was far too weak for any kind of decent fight, and all I had was a small pocket knife instead of a sweet sword . . . that fight would be a joke and I would lose miserably. I just prayed they would leave me alone. About that time, I remembered I had an antacid tablet and decided to eat that in some hope of soothing my very upset stomach. I ate it, and realized I probably shouldn't have eaten anything because it triggered some sort of evacuation button in my stomach that meant that it was coming back with a vengeance. I jumped out of the tent hoping the coyotes weren't there to greet me just in time for a gushing fire hose type barf to fly out my mouth. The noise I made I guess was far more terrifying than the coyotes had ever heard because I heard them scampering off while I laughed to myself at the amount that was coming out of my body. Throwing up and laughing is an incredibly strange feeling. It was far from proportional to the size of an antacid tablet. That was the last big barf-sesh: 4:55 am.

CHAPTER 69

Crawling back into the tent, I was cold, shaken, tired, still wet, and scared. I only heard from the coyotes one more time, and it was about 10 minutes after I crawled back in my tent and they were howling very far away from me. At 5:30 am my phone rang. Through blurry eyes I looked at the phone to see my friend, Adam's picture on it. Needless to say, I was very confused, and wasn't actually sure if he was really calling or if I was really losing it.

I answered the phone, "Hello? Adam?"

"Dude! How's it going!?"

"Um, good?"

"Oh man, did I wake you up?"

"Nah, I've been up, I've got a bit of food poisoning."

"Oh man!! That sucks! Except, it's just not quite crossing the country under your own power if you don't have food poisoning at some point."

Adam had ridden his bike across the country from Oregon to Virginia in 45 days just last summer; a trip that he, too, had gotten food poisoning on.

I laughed, "Yea, man, I guess you're right. It's rough. What are you doing up at this time anyway?" It was 4:30 his time.

"It's our spring break, we're all hiking. It sucks! There is snow up to our waist and it is freezing! I thought I'd call to check in while I had some service up here."

"Believe it or not, I would love to be out there with you guys. This trip is turning out to be tough."

"But you're doing it, man! You are more than halfway across a country, and you ran it. You can do it, not that you'd stop even if you wanted to."

"Thanks dude, I appreciate it."

We talked for a little bit longer, but decided we should both save our cell phone batteries in case we needed them for later. His call could not have come at a better time. I decided to pack up my stuff and get an early start on my way to Lake Village. I knew I would be walking the majority of it for a couple reasons. The first being I had no energy in my body and I had no way of getting calories into me without them being thrown violently from my system soon after consuming them. The second is that even if I could run, I doubt my stomach could handle the shaking and motion without some pretty devastating repercussions. I had to cover the 23 miles by 3 o'clock but since I would have to walk most of it, I might be cutting it close.

As I packed up my stuff, my fingers were so cold from the tent that was wet with frosty dew. I couldn't fold my tent so I ended up shoving everything into the jogger and decided to fix it when I got there. I made my way down the road on weak legs that seemed to quiver as I moved. I tried to walk as fast as I could for hopes of warm blood flowing, but got very tired very quickly. Between one of my trips out of the tent last night, I had written an email to my parents just in case something happened and they didn't hear from me, they would know what happened. My mom must have just read the email because I got a call from her. It was nice to talk to someone, especially my mom, as I walked down the road in the early morning chill. The exact details of the conversation were blurred by stomach aches, wobbly legs, and a dizzy head. My head pounded with a ferocious headache most likely due to dehydration.

The phone call started with a detailed description of my night from hell. And then it shifted the way my mom made a habit of doing throughout the trip. She helped ease my pain by distracting me with other things. Topics of home, and what my siblings had been up to lately, my sister's latest animal printed fashions, and my brother's latest obsessions. By the end of our conversation, I was starting to feel warmer, and slightly stronger.

Before long, I came to a very tiny town. It was a total of about 1 mile long and at the far eastern side of town there was a little convenience store. Since I had no calories in my system, and I hadn't gotten sick in a few hours at this point, I decided I should try to get some liquid calories in my system to kick start some energy. I walked in and grabbed two Mountain Dews. At 290 calories per bottle, it was just what the doctor ordered: carbonation to help settle my stomach, and sheer unadulterated calories for my energy levels, plus some caffeine just for fun. I drank the first one rather quickly because it was crisp and cold, even though it tasted kind of funny which I just attributed to barfing all night. After drinking the whole thing I looked at the bottle before throwing it away and noticed it had expired about 6 months prior. Since nothing seemed to happen, and I didn't even know Mountain Dew could expire, I decided to drink the other one too, even though it had technically expired three months before the first one I drank which brought that bottle to a whopping 9 months expired.

I was surprised at how quickly my systems turned on and how good I was feeling after drinking both bottles. The pace of my walk picked up, and I was even able to pepper in a little bit of running, though it wasn't much, simply because I was very tired. While walking down a particularly long straight stretch of road, a car pulled up next to me. A man stuck his head out the window and said, "Hey son, how ya doin today?"

I looked at the man and realized it was the last person I had talked to the day before; the same guy that I had hoped would invite me into his house. I replied with a simple, "Good, how are you?"

"Good, good, how did the camping work out?"

I didn't want to tell him the whole story of being wet and cold, being sick, and terrified; so again, I responded, "Good."

"Alrighty then, be safe!" And the man drove away. While I never actually stopped moving to talk to him that day, I wasn't mad at him, and didn't hold it against him for not inviting me in. There was a small part of me that didn't understand why I wasn't angry with him, but a larger part of me was glad he didn't have me come in. Besides, being that sick in someone's house that I just met would have been incredibly awkward, so I am glad I did not subject them to some of the noises I made.

By the end of the day I was able to run consistently for about a mile and then needed a walking break. It was just too exhausting. Huge flat fields with nothing presently in them accompanied me on my trek that day, and would provide my scenery. Many small creeks with bridges no longer than 20 feet littered my route as I came closer and closer to the great Mississippi River. I passed by the schools for Lake Village as I approached the town. When I came within about a mile and a half of where I was supposed to be ending that day a police car pulled up and the officer rolled down the window to the Dodge Charger painted black and white.

"I'm guessing you're Patrick McGlade."

"Yes, sir . . ."

"Welcome to Lake Village, there is a light up ahead, please follow me and I'll show you where you're going."

It was a police escort! Another car pulled up so I had one car in front of me and another one behind me. I was stoked, but that meant that I had to run, because I'm sure he didn't want to drive any slower than I could run. I picked up the pace and cruised on through the light chasing the police car, and running away from the other. We cruised down the main street and passed the restaurant, Rhoda's Famous Hot Tamales. Most of the time, when I entered a town, I might get a few strange looks, but was pretty well under the radar. Not today; the police cars had their lights on, and would turn on the siren for just a second so it would make the *whoop* sound but not go through the whole siren cycle, drawing lots of attention to us. People stared, but didn't really do anything but stare. We turned left when we got to Lake Chicot and ended shortly after that, in front of town hall.

I thanked the officers for driving with me and several people came out of town hall. I was so tired I had to find a bench to sit down. The last stretch of that day with the police escort was the furthest I had run all day and now I felt sick and my head spun like crazy. I felt terrible while I was meeting people and tried very hard to be pleasant but I was pretty sure I was going to barf and smelled terrible. There was a plan to have refreshments, and for a couple of people to come meet me there. I had gotten there about an hour and a half early though, so no one was expecting me yet, which was nice because I was able to regroup and figure out a way not to barf in front of a ton of people I hadn't met. Brianne, the woman who we had been in contact with for the town of Lake Village, came up and introduced herself.

Brianne was very welcoming and incredibly nice. She was petite with long light brown hair, and though she had more energy than a Chihuahua after drinking several cups of coffee, she wasn't obnoxious by any stretch of the imagination. Due to her enthusiasm, organization skill, and general stoked-ness for her job and the run, I had guessed that she would have been a little older than the mid to late 20s that she was. She had a broad smile and incredibly straight, white teeth. It wasn't that I was expecting otherwise, but they were the kind of teeth you see in the dentist office magazines.

We had some time before I was actually supposed to start meeting people so a reporter took me across the square to the newspaper's office so we could do an interview. Soon after that, I made my way back over to the town hall where there were several people waiting along with the local private school in town, St. Mary's. After sharing a few brief words with all of them and taking a few pictures, Brianne offered to show me where she lived so I could take a shower while she finished up some of her work. While the walk to her house was no more than about half a mile, it seemed like it took forever because I was so exhausted both physically and mentally from the previous nights' *activities*. Since Lake Village wasn't very big, she was able to point out some pretty key buildings in the town and give me a little tour on the way.

After arriving and showering, I flopped down on the bed I was being lent just to regroup until her friends came over for pizza that night. It was a good thing I had a little bit of time because I promptly fell asleep in a semi-coma. When I awoke a little later, I was very confused of my whereabouts because it was dark out. But being winter, it was only about 6 o'clock. Before long, some of Brianne's friends came over. They were an interesting bunch. Most of them were not much older than I was, and none of them over 30. They were all brought to Lake Village for the Teach for America program. Teach for America is a program where brand new teachers join the "corps" and are placed in either an urban or rural low-income area where the kids do not have the same opportunities as other areas of the country. They sign up for a two year commitment and after talking to them all, I realize how difficult this task truly is. Most of the kids they taught have never been outside of Lake Village and they don't have the opportunity for a good education and these young teachers are out there to hopefully change that. Besides being on a mission, they were all really nice and pretty funny too. The pizza was delicious, the company was great, and I was inside a house. Things had definitely turned around since last night.

CHAPTER 70

The next day's events started with a car ride out to the Mississippi River Bridge. The spot where I would be crossing actually had two bridges; an old one, and a new one. The new one wasn't open to traffic yet, but the old was very small. Despite being very old, there was a certain air about the old one that made my decision of which bridge to run over a little bit difficult. See, in the movie Forrest Gump, he ran over the old one and since I had started planning this trip, that had seemed to be a nickname that was used a lot. We weren't sure which one I would be allowed to cross, so I decided not to spend too much time worrying about which bridge to run over.

The reason we went out to the bridge that day, though, was because the man who was riding a buggy pulled by his horse all around the country was planning on crossing the Mississippi River that day. I had heard about him back in Strong, when I camped at Medlin's Hardware, but it seemed that I had caught up to him. Brianne and I pulled up to the new bridge and waited for the mayor and a police officer to escort him over the new bridge. It looked like I would be able to run on the new one after all. We waited there for awhile and then decided to drive over to the Mississippi side of the bridge to see if he was over there. Sure enough, as we pulled up, we saw a big covered wagon being pulled by a horse moseying down the other side of the bridge heading east into Mississippi.

We pulled ahead of him and waited. He seemed to be in no hurry at all. I was fascinated by his home on wheels. It was very different than a motor home, and far different than anything else I had seen. Its base was a car chassis and he had built the rest of the wooden wagon on top of the chassis. Everything else inside was made of wood, and the covering for the top was a giant blue tarp. I'm sure that worked better in keeping out the rain than a cloth covering would. We walked next to him and the news reporter asked him questions.

The man was from Corpus Christi, Texas. Gray hair and gray beard, slightly rotund, and was wearing overalls. He had a dog sitting in his lap. The man had been on the road for a year and a half! More than a year, and he was just now crossing the Mississippi River. I couldn't imagine the patience that must take. He had an interesting take on life, and the reason he was doing it. It wasn't for charity or because his wife kicked him out of the house. He hadn't won the lottery, and he didn't get fired from his job. This wasn't a mid-life crisis, or a protest, or an attempt at any record. He didn't have a slogan or website, and as far as I know, he wasn't charging massive amounts of electronics in the back of his wagon. The man who appeared to be in his late 60s-early 70s just wanted to see the country before he got old, and 3 miles an hour, to him, was the perfect speed to do it.

"Before I get old."

Those words resonated in my head for the rest of the day; and still resonate in my head. I was 21 years old. And here was a man who was much older than 50 and was achieving his dream before he "got old." This guy truly lived by the "seize the day" mentality, and he was doing what he wanted to do. Listening to his responses to the interviewer's questions, I realized that this guy didn't want to be bothered with questions of why, or when he will return home, or where he is going next. He didn't know the answer to the questions, and he didn't care to have them answered. He was completely happy and quite content just being. Sitting on the bench in his wagon, with the reigns of his horse in one hand a miniature dog in the other, gave him enough sanity to live on.

After watching him plod on down the road, we made our way to the school where I would speak with two classes. But first, we stopped by Rhoda's Famous Hot Tamales. The restaurant was a tiny little place with a big glass container where you could point out what you wanted the feast to come with. When we walked in there was a woman behind the counter who was taking orders and generally socializing with everyone in the restaurant. She was very nice but didn't move very fast. This wasn't a problem because we were in no hurry, but I did find it a little bit strange because any place I had ever been had treated the speed of the service as something that was important.

Later, Brianne informed me that sometimes things just move a little bit slower in the south. It has nothing to do with "bad service" and it's not because they don't care, they just value personal relationships more than the "get in and get out" mentality that a lot of places have. They expect you to hang out, talk for awhile, and just chill.

After we finished ordering, Brianne said to the lady behind the counter, "Hey, guess what he's doing?"

The lady looked at her puzzled and then looked at me like I should have had a third eyeball and replied, "What?"

"He is running across the whole country, California to Georgia."

"The whole country? Mmm . . . Boy, you crazy!"

Then she turned toward an older lady sitting at one of the tables in the restaurant and yelled, "Ay Rhoda! This boy's running across the country!"

The incredibly petite lady turned toward us and she started asking me questions about it. I found it pretty cool to meet the famous Rhoda.

Following the tamales, which were incredibly tasty by the way, we made our way over to the school where Brianne's friends taught. The kids there were like none I had ever met. Most of them had never been out of that town and were hardly exposed to anything like running "for fun" or running across a country. Their teacher, Daniel, was a biker and did some running and he told me that if any of his students ever saw him out for a run they'd ask what he was running from. Even as high school kids, they didn't know much about the running community but they sure knew about sprinting. They had a track team and a football team. Running outside of that was foreign. When I showed them my packets of Gu they were taken aback and one kid wanted to try it. Everyone else just stared at him while Daniel tore off the top and squeezed a little bit of the Vanilla flavored Gu onto his finger. When he saw what it looked like he made a face but then ate it anyway. A bunch of the girls in the class started laughing and looked away, but the other guys in the class were interested in his take on being the first in the class to give the syrupy liquid a try. He gave a couple of funny looks while he was deciding on how it tasted, then without saying anything nodded his head with approval and several more hands shot up so they could try it too. Most didn't like it, but some asked where they could get their own.

They also asked several questions, my favorite being, "When you get to a lake or river, do you swim across it?"

After that, Brianne took me to Lake Port Plantation which was a really great old house from the days of the cotton plantations. Everything about the house was huge. The ceilings were tall, the doors were 10 or 12 feet tall, and the base boards were very wide.

The people who were in charge of the house were working on restoration with some college students.

The last thing in the town I hadn't seen up close and personal was Lake Chicot. Luckily, Brianne was way ahead of me on that one and at the north end of the lake they have a park where they give boat tours. The tour guide had a great sense of humor and knew way more than the average person about birds. So, like any good tour guide, she passed much of her knowledge onto us. Unfortunately, I don't remember any of it—there was just too much.

I had talked to a runner named Wally who said that he wanted to run over the bridge with me and said he might be bringing a friend. I had no opposition and really looked forward to running with anyone for any amount of time. Since I would be meeting with a couple people to run over the Mississippi River Bridge the next day, I wanted to get a good night's sleep.

CHAPTER 71

I woke up the following morning and started running the 9 or 10 miles to the foot of the Mississippi River Bridge. When I came around the last bend in the road, I saw a crowd of people gathered at the start of the bridge in the same area Brianne and I had waited for the horse and carriage the previous day. As I got closer I was able to count 7 people who were dressed in running clothes. Very surprised at the gathering of runners, I greeted them and thanked them for all coming. We stood around for a little while just talking and waiting for the police to come down to the bridge so we could have an escort. Once they came we realized we needed the key to open the gate that blocked them. After some more waiting, we were able to start.

The ages of the runners ranged from 30 to 70 and everyone was excited to be there. We all ran in a straight line side by side. Running with this many people gave the crossing something extra. Crossing the Mississippi River was a big deal for the development of our country. It's really a massive river. The famed stretch of water was the subject of many songs, stories, and legends. I was now crossing this famous river and would be happily running *east of the Mississippi* from here on out.

After the three mile bridge, I thanked everyone for coming. We snapped a picture next to the welcome sign for the state of Mississippi. Then, I made my way down the road toward the first town in Mississippi.

After running for about 20 minutes a beat up car stopped and asked if I was Patrick McGlade. He was a reporter for a local newspaper. The man pulled his beat up car over to the side of the road and opened his door. Lots of trash fell out of the car as he did a sort of roll maneuver and stumbled toward me. I got the hint he'd partied pretty hard the night before and the effects of whatever alcoholic beverage he had chosen still hadn't worn off.

When he reached my side of the road he started talking and his breath smelled like he had just finished a 12 pack in the previous 5 minutes.

He opened with, "Man, I'm not even supposed to be working right now, I was right in the middle of hanging with my boy."

I'm not sure whether he meant his friend or son.

I simply responded, "Bummer."

"Yea no kidding dude. So what are you doing anyway?"

I told him what I was doing in the fewest amount of words possible just so I could continue on toward the next town of Hollondale.

He responded with, "Well, I guess that covers it. Good luck."

With that, he stumbled back to his car climbed back in and sped off. I wasn't sure if that story would ever get written or published, but that day I wasn't too concerned with it. I was very tired and the road was flatter than I had ever seen.

The farmland that spread out on each side of the road was just flat dirt. There wasn't a plant to be seen; just dust. When even the slightest breeze picked up it would start mini-twisters of dust. I only hoped that they wouldn't come around me. After coming to the end of a particularly straight portion of road, I had a choice: turn left, or go straight and walk up on the levee of the Mississippi River. I figured since I would more than likely never be in this spot in the country again, I should take every opportunity I could to do something I couldn't do again.

I pushed my jogger up the steep grassy side of the levee and found that there was gravel on top. This made running with the jogger near impossible so I decided to walk. It was very nice up there. Since it was the highest point around, I could see pretty far into the distance. I walked along and enjoyed the views of the flat Mississippi delta region.

After several miles of walking along the top of the levee, I finally noticed a road off to the side that I knew from the maps as the road I should be on. I came down off the levee and continued on roads. Several miles later, the back country road I was on turned into gravel again and so I walked. The pattern of gravel, dirt road, and slightly paved road continued for the rest of the day. While the road never rose or fell unless there was a bridge, more and more foliage appeared and would then fall away on the sides of the road to open into farmland. When I finally did get to Hollondale, I was utterly exhausted and debated not even eating dinner and just going to sleep. Luckily, my stomach won that argument and I ate first.

CHAPTER 72

The next morning I woke up and since I wasn't meeting anyone but was staying in a hotel that night I took my time and just relaxed for much of the morning and caught up on rest. I still hadn't been sleeping well as of late. Every now and then, the lack of sleep would catch up to me and I would crash hard. When I finally did awake, I looked out the window and saw that it was very overcast and windy. It looked cold outside. My motivation to pack up and go outside plummeted. Since I really had no choice I layered myself well, packed up the jogger and opened the door. It was snowing very heavily but was not sticking to the ground. Excited to see snow, I closed the door and put on my jacket and long pants. When I opened the door again, less than 2 minutes later, it was not snowing a single flake. Slightly confused I closed the door and took off the jacket and long pants thinking that shorts would be fine, as long as my legs didn't get wet.

When I opened the door again, it wasn't snowing which I was somewhat glad to see because I had just removed my snow/rain clothes. As I made my way across the parking lot of the hotel I had stayed at I realized that today's weather would be truly unpleasant. Cold and windy.

Running down the road, I passed an incredible amount of ponds. They were all about the same size, square or rectangle and full of catfish. They were all catfish farms. The wind whipped across the small bodies of water and in some cases, carried with it spray from the water. Luckily it didn't smell like fish. The cold and windy weather only got more miserable when the wind would shift for a few minutes and there would be a sleet downpour. The tiny frozen rain drops pelted the backs of my ears and stung me. Then the wind would shift again and the ice balls would pound the side of my face and fly into my ears for a little while. And then, as quickly as it started, it ended. It was just an off and on strange weather pattern all day.

CHAPTER 73

The following day, I exited the delta region.

A couple of days before I crossed the Mississippi River, the hills disappeared. Now, a couple of days after I had crossed the Mississippi River, the hills were still nowhere to be found. It got somewhat monotonous and made the miles crawl by. With no hills in the distance to mark the distance that I could cross off my pile of miles left, I soon became tired of the flatness.

Seemingly out-of-nowhere, I turned a corner and saw the road curve upward about a mile and a half to two miles down the road. I could have sworn that I was mistaken because I couldn't imagine the land so suddenly making such a drastic change in topography.

As I ran further, I soon realized it wasn't a mistake and all the cars were climbing the road leaving the delta. From a ways back it looked like an anthill but as I watched the cars climb this thing, I soon realized it was a very large anthill, and quite steep as well. When I reached the bottom of the long straight hill I looked to each side and sure enough, the land formed a sort of shelf that just decided that it would start to curve up from here. I found the severity and suddenness of change absolutely fascinating.

I needed to keep going and as I started running up the hill I was forced to walk up a hill for the first time in almost a week. It was very steep. Soon, even holding a pace of a fast walk, while pushing the stroller, became difficult. The road continued to climb, and became curvy making it increasingly more dangerous as the shoulder fell away to reveal large ditches and drops. Upon reaching the top I noticed that the topography was not the only thing that had changed suddenly. The vegetation growth had become very thick and lush.

And a plant I had never seen before displayed itself as it lay dormant covering an entire field in its vast network of curling and spiraling vines.

Kudzu is technically a weed and it grows throughout the southeast. It grows incredibly fast; as much as a foot per day in the summer months. The plant crawls up trees, telephone poles, even cars; and swallows them. I later learned that it is not a native plant. It was a gift from the Japanese and was initially thought of as a great idea because it grows so fast and greatly helps to control erosion. When it first arrived, people planted it like crazy and the government helped support its growth, and then soon realized it was swallowing the south. Now, it covers approximately 7 million acres of the Deep South. I also learned that one way to get rid of it is to have goats come in and eat it. After they have eaten all they can, bring boars in and they will dig up the roots and eat those. I heard mixed reviews on the residents' of the south's love or hate for the plant, some love; some hate, but most dislike it.

After reaching Lexington's limits, I found the motel I was staying in that night. It was donated by a family much like many rooms before that one. The motel itself was slightly sketchy looking and mostly run down, but I didn't mind. I went into the office and spoke with the owner.

The owner told me I was a huge hassle because someone had called to tell him I was coming and tried to pay for the room in advance, and they were very insistent so he finally gave in even though it was "clearly" against policy to reserve rooms, as it was obviously stated in magic marker on the cardboard sign in his window. I apologized for his inconvenience but thanked him for making me an exception. He didn't reply. He just slid me the keys and remote for the TV and pointed in the direction of my room without saying another word.

When I reached the room, I jimmied the key in the doorknob until it unlocked. I was greeted by a puke green room, a light pink bedspread and a 10 ft x 10 ft mirror covering most of the far wall. I couldn't imagine someone needed a mirror that big but hey, there are some large people in the world.

After showering, my stomach growled, which meant it was feeding time. I checked my phone for the local pizza joint and called with an order, large Hawaiian with peppers, mushrooms, onions and pepperoni. I was stoked. Just saying the ingredients out loud made my mouth water. Unfortunately they did not deliver so I asked the lady on the phone where they were located in reference to my hotel. "Right around the corner." Bonus.

I put on my shoes and started walking. Phone in hand with the address, I was following the directions my gadget fed me. After walking about a mile, it led me to a spot in the road that clearly had no pizza place around it. I didn't really know what to do so I started to call the pizza place back.

As I put the phone up to my ear, a car pulled up and a middle aged guy dressed in camouflage rolled down his window and said, "Hey! I'm going to need you to get in the car now."

I looked at him trying not to laugh. Did this guy really expect me to just say, *Oh okay,* and get in his car?

Although, when I looked at him he looked scared. And I didn't think it was the kind of scared where he wasn't really, it's just how his face looked. He looked genuinely scared.

I said, "Excuse me?"

"I really need you to get in the car now . . . please. You aren't from around here, are you?"

For some reason, even though the guy was easily a foot taller than me and was about double my width. I didn't get the feeling this guy was trying to abduct me.

I answered with, "Um . . . okay."

I walked around the back of his car and opened the passenger side door. He was clearing off the seat and throwing things into the back seat frantically like I needed to get in as soon as I possibly could.

After getting in and closing the door he said, "Look man, I'm really sorry about this . . ." Immediately I thought, *Oh great, he seemed okay, but now that I'm in his car he's 'sorry' for something. I did just get abducted.*

He continued, "You are walking around a *really* bad part of town. What are you doing here? Do you not have a car?"

I told him, "I just ordered a pizza and since I'm running across the country and they didn't deliver I had to go pick it up this way but I didn't expect it to be this far."

We got to a light and he did a U-turn. "Wait . . . what? You're running across the country?" "Yes, and I'm staying in the motel near the sign for the town but the pizza place is supposed to be somewhere around here but I don't know where."

We kept driving further and further away from the motel.

"Geeze, man, that's awesome. How about I just drive you to get your pizza and give you a ride back to the motel?"

"Wow! That'd be awesome. Thank you!"

We pulled up to the pizza place and I jumped out, went in and when I came out I half expected him to be gone, but he wasn't.

I got back in the car and he wafted the steaming pizza smell to his nose and gave me a look that said, "Good choice, you've done well grasshopper."

He was on the phone with his wife and was telling her why he'd be a little late.

After he got off the phone I offered him a slice or two but he said he thought I might need it a little bit more than he would. When we reached the motel he gave me his phone number in case I needed anything. He told me as soon as I get in the door, lock it, and do not come out until morning. "Tomorrow morning you should be alright because I'm assuming you'll be leaving decently early."

I thanked him profusely for helping me and driving me around and as quickly as he had appeared, he drove off and I haven't heard from him since.

When I got in the room I started chowing down on the pizza and opened the book I was reading but couldn't really focus on what I was reading. That experience was too weird. After thinking about it for awhile I thought there were several things that were very strange about what had happened that evening. But perhaps the strangest was how comfortable I was with getting in a complete stranger's car and it turning out to be okay. Normally this thought would give someone the willies, but I guess that's what my dad was talking about when he told me, "Listen to the little voice, it's usually right."

CHAPTER 74

The day I ran into the town of Kosciusko (pronounced Koziesco) I started nice and early. I enjoyed running in the cool early morning. It was incredibly humid, but since it was pretty cool outside, there seemed to be a mist that floated delicately above the ground. Dew-covered spider webs seemed to sparkle as the barely risen sun shined on them through trees that were just starting to sprout leaves. The fields on either side of the road gave off a purplish and orange glow that was incredibly soothing while my breathing and foot strikes were the only things that made any noise.

As the morning crept on, more and more cars appeared and school busses flew by always bringing with them a giant gust of wind that would've woke me up had I still been asleep. I ran over short bridges with streams underneath and around blind curves that always seemed to bring with it more cars. I passed through tiny towns where I was sure not to blink because they were gone before I had run another quarter mile.

Though it was a shorter running day in terms of mileage, it was a very relaxing day. Most of my running was done before it got warm and I was able to watch the sun come up. I met JP at a gas station in Kosciusko. He had offered me a place to stay and a ride to and from the pick-up point, but other than that, I had no idea how he heard of the run or his relation to the run. I had talked to him on the phone the night before to coordinate a meeting place and picked up on his deep southern drawl. I approached the truck that he said he would be in and a thin, fit looking man with short brown hair and a scraggly beard stepped out. He looked very friendly as he smiled and I could tell he was some sort of athlete himself. His cheeks had the "endurance runner's hollow" as my mom's friend puts it and you could see it even under his scruffy beard.

We loaded my stuff into the bed of his truck and started off toward his house. He was incredibly friendly and told me about his family. His two high school aged daughters were still in school but I would meet them later along with his wife. He told me about the area we were in and revealed that he is in the timber business. He explained that it entailed going out in the woods and hiking while scoping a tree farmer's land so they could harvest their trees. I also found out that he learned about the run from his running group.

He was a runner himself, as I had suspected, and ran any distance he could get his hands on, though he said that recently he had preferred the shorter road races. During those, he was able to push a little kid in a wheel chair, who was even more competitive than JP was, and always wanted to win. JP usually ran very well and had won his age group in several races but unfortunately, the little boy didn't get the concept of age group winners and was usually disappointed with their standings.

While showing me around the area we stopped in for a bite to eat at an old drug store. They make a killer turkey sandwich and an even better vanilla milkshake. The Neshoba Fair Grounds are a place where people gather every summer . . . though, that might be the understatement of the century. Let me just start off by saying it's a place like no other. Before visiting it, I would have never been able to picture it had someone described it to me. JP told me about a giant fair they have every year that never stops. It is coined as *Mississippi's house party*.

When we pulled up to the gates it looked like a ghost town, and that's essentially what it is most weeks of the year. The first thing you notice when you pull up are tons and tons of brightly and oddly painted cabins that look more like 3 stories of tree house than cabins where people live comfortably. The "roads," which were closer in species to alleys, were dirt and the cabins were so close together they looked like medieval town houses. It didn't look like a very well planned space. JP informed me that it wasn't planned at all. It started as a church, community, and agricultural fair in 1889. People would come and park their wagons in a circle and camp out for the duration of the fair. Little by little the fair grew and soon cabins replaced wagons and a horse track was built in the "town's" center. As the fair grew, so did the number of cabins. They just built them wherever there was space. Because of this, they weren't planned in a normal city-plan sort of way.

Strings of lights still hung and when they swayed in the breeze it made the lack of people an even more eerie sight. We got out of the truck and decided to walk around. In a sort of town square there was a stage underneath a roof with lots of wooden benches. Bands came and played during the summer to help entertain the masses of people. Nowadays there are over 600 cabins and a lot for 200 RVs. JP said during the days of the fair there is a line of cars that goes for miles outside the campground waiting to get in. And there are parties going on 24 hours a day. Lots of people use it as a place for reunions. Family and friends gather and pack the cabins full to the brim. It sounded slightly nutty, very quirky, and like a pretty fun way to spend a week in the summer.

By the time we had explored the empty town that was the Neshoba County fairgrounds, the girls were getting out of school. We made our way to his house where we picked up his kayaks and his oldest daughter, Hannah, so we could go float on the Pearl River. Kayaking was very relaxing and it was great to be in the woods. I really missed that about trail running. If this was the closest I could get to being in the woods, then that would be just fine. Cypress trees grew in the water and their huge roots exposed themselves in a very eerie way. When you're used to seeing something it's not as big of a deal, so I was way more fascinated with these trees than I think JP or Hannah was.

At one point during the float, JP, sitting behind me in a two-man kayak, pointed at an overhanging tree branch with his oar. Curled and semi draped across the branch was a cotton mouth snake that looked like it had the same circumference as a baseball. He said, "Oh man, that's the biggest I've seen! You want to get a picture with it?" Since I'm really not a fan of snakes I declined his generous offer but asked about it because as far as I knew, we didn't have any cotton mouths in Virginia.

"Oh, they're a nasty snake. They'll just sit there waiting for you to get closer and closer. They aren't afraid of you and right before they strike they open their mouth all the way and it looks like they've got cotton balls in their mouth. Hence, cotton mouth." I was happy that I had declined his offer to take a picture with the snake at that point.

After we finished the float, we returned to the house. JP went immediately to work cooking dinner while I met and visited with JP's wife, Sewanna, and other daughter Rebekah. Since I was burning so many calories per day, he decided that I needed to eat bacon that night. I had no objection. We had cheese stuffed chicken wrapped in bacon and jalapenos with cream cheese stuffed inside of them. He also had some friends come over. Joey had a smile on his face from the time he entered the house until he left that night. He was a little bit stockier than JP was and looked like he could also handle himself in a boxing match as well as running. Ultra marathons have a wider variety of body types displayed in them, and Joey was here to prove it. He had completed a couple of 50 milers but his ultimate goal was the Barkley Marathon, which is more like a survival than a race.

There are no course markings and most of the time no trail. A racer must rip a page out of 12 books on the course to prove they completed each lap. 5 laps of 20 miles is the goal of each starter and each loop has 11,820 ft of elevation gain and 11,820 ft of elevation loss making the whole race a grand total of 59,100 feet of elevation gain and loss. And yes, that is like climbing Everest . . . twice. Only eleven people have ever finished since the first race in 1986. Most drop out after the first lap; and Joey wanted to do it. He said he was more worried about the distance and elevation part of the run than the orienteering. The race time is never announced in advance and the race fee is an old license plate. Needless to say, we talked much about that.

JP's friends, Jacob and Kimberly, also came for dinner. They were around my age and were both great people to hang out with. We all sat outside in the cool evening and enjoyed the great bacon wrapped food and sweet tea, which I still enjoyed.

CHAPTER 75

Several weeks before I ran into Louisville, Mississippi, I received an email from a man named Mike Forster telling me about his granddaughter. He was excited that I was coming through his town of Louisville offered me a place to stay. As soon as I accepted, he went to work planning my stay there. I had a scheduled day off there and as plans started to unfold, it looked like a second day off in Louisville was going to be needed.

He had plans for me to speak to several schools, dinners, lunches, radio interviews, and more. Though he told me about it all before I got there, it turned out to be even bigger than I thought. And it all started before I even arrived.

The morning I was to run into Louisville I woke up at JP's house and got ready to go. I wanted to start nice and early because I had a time that I absolutely had to be in Louisville to meet Mike. As soon as I started, so did the rain. It was very chilly. I even had my headlamp on to help me stay visible. No more than an hour after the rain started, it stopped and I was left to run the rest of the day in my wet shoes. The humidity was insane when the soaked streets began to dry out. JP told me about a back road that would be a lot prettier and much safer to run on than the main road; and he was right. I meandered through the trees and the wet evergreen timber smelled like Christmas trees. The lack of cars was very calming and the only sounds I heard were of birds chirping while taking their early morning baths. The very familiar rhythm of my feet and breathing weaved themselves together with the quiet slick sound of the tires rolling along the newly wet streets. The few houses on this road were tucked back in the trees and sometimes barely visible to me; certainly not visible to anyone in a car driving past. I have a feeling they wanted it that way.

After my little back road hike, I turned left on a more populated road, yet still very quiet with one car passing me every 5 to 10 minutes at speeds that I expected to get a sonic boom out of. The lack of shoulder would have made this road far more dangerous had it been more heavily populated. Timber trucks passed me spraying wood chips and pieces of bark that annoyingly got stuck to my sweaty skin. As I continued down the road, I realized I had been moving at a fairly quick pace and would arrive two hours before I was supposed to. I stopped running and just walked. I really took my time and enjoyed being in such a green area. After I was certain the rain had stopped for the day, I stopped and changed my socks and put on a fresh shirt.

Not too long after I decided that I could run again without being too far ahead, I got a phone call saying that two runners were going to run the last 10 miles into the town with me. They were on their way out driving with Mike.

I didn't know what kind of car I was looking for, but I figured when a car slowed down with three men inside, it must be them. Mike was in the driver's seat of his convertible, Brian in the passenger seat, and Bubba in the back. The top was down because it had turned into such a nice day. Mike pulled the car off the road and immediately got out. I had spoken with him several times through email, and a time or two on the phone but this was the first time I met him in person. He was smiling from ear to ear when he got out of the car and came to shake my hand. I knew he was old enough to be a grandfather, but I guessed he couldn't be any older than mid 60's. He sported the same haircut as my own grandpa, stood about 5' 7" and wore glasses. He was wearing a polo shirt and shorts and had a very confident air about him.

"It's nice to finally meet you in person, Patrick." He spoke deliberately, annunciated perfectly, and had a very slight, sophisticated southern drawl to his voice.

"Nice to meet you too, Mr. Forster." I responded.

He gave me the plan of the next 10 miles, and what would happen when I got to the first intersection in town. Afterwards he got back in his convertible, and sped off down the road.

I loved the company of Bubba and Brian. Both were long distance runners and both were quite fast. Brian was a bit older than Bubba and shorter and thinner too. He looked like he had been running since high school, and truly enjoyed it. He had great running form. Bubba, couldn't have been older than

30 and had a more muscular frame. Even with a bigger body, he seemed to run effortlessly. Being in the company of two fresh runners gave me some added energy, as I was not feeling very well at this point.

We passed a couple of giant bulls in the pasture off to the left side of the road. These bulls were humungous and they looked mad. Giant horns jutted out of each side of their skulls and they looked like they weighted multiple tons. They informed me that those bulls were used for rodeos. We passed the time asking each other questions, and getting to know each other. They were really great guys, had an awesome sense of humor, and I was glad to get the chance to run with them.

The main road coming in from the west goes down a hill, so you can see a good distance ahead without anything blocking your view of the first part of the town. At the bottom of the hill there is a stop light where I saw a news crew on the side of the road and police cars ready to turn on their lights and block the intersection. At the gas station right after the light there were two fire trucks waiting for us. Amanda and Rebecca were in one of the trucks with giant smiles on their faces. About where the police cars were, just before the light, there were also three high school kids that wanted to run the last two miles into town to city hall with us. We welcomed the company and resumed running into the town of Louisville.

CHAPTER 76

Now with one police car in front of us, and two fire trucks and police car behind us, the 6 of us ran down the road knowing that we were the cause of some traffic and the sirens were making quite a bit of noise. We ran up the last hill before the town. None of us really knew where we were supposed to be going, so we followed the police car when it turned right and ended up right where we were supposed to: on the steps of city hall.

I was very surprised at the amount of people that had come out to support the run. Not only did 5 runners come out to finish the day with me, but all of city hall workers seemed to pour out onto the street, along with the news team, various people from the town and the preschool from the church across the street were sitting on the stairs of the church holding signs that said, "Run Patrick Run."

It was really quite a sight. Amid all of the handshakes and introductions, camera flashes and people talking I heard the kids across the street chanting "Run Patrick Run." The whole scene reminded me of a dream where I'm the center of attention and then I realize I'm naked or have a huge booger hanging out of my nose.

I didn't really know what I was supposed to do but a news reporter came over with a giant camera. He didn't introduce himself. He just said, "Why are you running?" I paused for a minute because the first thing that popped into my head was the famous Forrest Gump quote, "I just felt like running!" I smiled, and gave my normal answer about kids with arthritis.

Thinking back, I wish I didn't have so much of a filter on my mouth. He probably would have found the Forrest Gump answer more humorous.

After another minute, Mike found me and brought me up to meet the mayor. It was then that he gave a few words, said some very nice things about me and presented me with a key to the city of Louisville, Mississippi. It was literally a giant, old fashioned key, painted gold and had "City of Louisville, MS" engraved on it.

That evening, more of Mike's family came over and we all had dinner together. It was absolutely delicious pulled barbeque chicken and pork.

Mike and Bette (pronounced like Betty) were the parents to Catherine Kuo (pronounced Kwoe, not Koo-oe) who was mother to Rebecca who had arthritis.

The following day was incredibly busy. It started at the radio station 107.1. Mike and Rebecca came with me, and Rebecca spoke on the radio. In reality, she seemed way more comfortable with it than I was. I had given several interviews since before I started the run and doing interviews were even still a little bit nerve wracking. Rebecca just sat down at the microphone and spoke like she had been doing it for years.

From the radio station we went to Mary Lou's Biscuit Bar for a famous sausage biscuit. The store was very small and they made all of their home-made biscuits right there in the shop. The walls were covered in signatures of people who had visited the shop. While looking at the walls I saw Ken Stannard's name. Ken had run across the country with two of his friends a couple years before I did and did almost the exact same route. I had talked with him before I left. He happened to be very helpful. Seeing his name on the wall made me think about people who would do the same route after me, and I wondered if they would come to the biscuit bar.

After devouring our sandwiches, we went to Winston Academy where I talked to the senior class. Louisville is a small town and Winston Academy is a private school so I was only talking to about 15-20 people. I liked the small group feel. They were right there in front of me and I could just talk like I was having a conversation instead of trying to talk as loud as I could to a large crowd. It was a great group of kids and they were genuinely interested, which was nice.

Upon leaving the school, we went to The Bypass Restaurant for lunch where they were doing a fund raiser for me. They were giving a percentage of the meals from 11am-2pm to the Arthritis Foundation. It was a great roadside family restaurant and had some killer salads. I would know.

The last stop of the day was Louisville High School to meet with their football team. This time the Kuo's came with us. School was just being let out and the football team filed into the locker room. I had some friends on the football team of my high school and none of them came anything close to the size of some of those guys walking through the door. Most of them were shaped like refrigerators. I firmly believe it would hurt less to be hit by a freight train than some of those players. Louisville was the state champion in 2009, and I'm sure they will be in the future as well.

After it was deemed "safe" for the girls we all entered the locker room and we were greeted by the standard locker room smell of sweat, feet, and dirt. I'm sure if I played football I would have loved that smell, but instead, it took a minute to get used to.

The coach introduced me and I started talking to them. They were all sitting scattered around the locker room so in order to see all of them I had to keep spinning. If I had thrown up while spinning, it might have made it as a skit on Saturday Night Live. Most of them never ran more the 100 yards at a time but a few of them were on the track team. I gave them the run-down of what I was doing. Most of their questions were related to the physical part of the run instead of the types of questions that the elementary schools asked such as where I went to the bathroom. They were very interested in my 40 yard dash time. Unfortunately I could not supply them with an answer.

The day ended with the pasta dinner fundraiser. This idea was fantastic and was held at the Presbyterian Church right in the middle of town. Everyone came together to donate the massive amount of food and sell tickets. I started out in the kitchen helping to cook piles of spaghetti and keep everything rolling until people started to arrive. Then I transitioned to talking with people who came to support the run. We had an incredible turnout and by the end of the evening our tally sheet read about 140 people. And between all of them, raised $2,500 dollars!

The kindness everyone showed was incredible. Their generosity was overwhelming. I was able to meet everyone there, and while I felt a bit like a politician, I was glad I was able speak with everyone. They were all so welcoming.

It's hard to explain how it feels to be welcomed like this, especially to a town you've never been to and have complete strangers come out of the woodwork to go above and beyond to help some "running nomad." It's the kind of thing that restores faith in humanity.

That night after the dinner and after everyone had gone to sleep I stared at the ceiling in the guest bedroom and thought about the fact that we had such a large crowd come out. Was it because there wasn't anything else to do that night? Possibly, but I'm pretty sure there was something on TV that they would have found entertaining if they didn't care about helping.

CHAPTER 77

The following day was another day off in Louisville, Mississippi. Mike decided it would be best to spend the day out in the woods at the Forsters' cabin. From the main road, we took a dirt road down to the Forsters' son's farm.

We got out and jumped the fence to play with the baby goats. They weren't very old, so they were absolutely terrified of us all. I learned the only way to catch a baby goat is to run it down; just chase it until you catch it. It sounds easy enough.

The funny thing about chasing goats, aside from the fact that you're chasing a baby goat, is that they sort of scream while they're being chased. They run around in circles trying to cut hard on their turns in an attempt to lose you while screaming. What's even funnier is every time a baby goat screamed; Amanda Kuo laughed her 4 year old laugh. Her giggle was enough to make anyone start laughing.

The chase lasted anywhere between 30 seconds to a minute and a half. It usually resulted in catching the little goats. I was surprised to feel how soft they were. The biggest, and most welcomed, surprise was that as babies, goats don't smell like their grown-up counterparts. They are just cute, non-smelly, screaming little goats.

After playing with the goats, we followed the road further back into the woods and through a gate. As we came around the last curve, a fairly large shed appeared with an antique gas pump near it. The cabin itself sat nestled back among the trees facing a small lake. It was absolutely beautiful. It was made entirely from logs. It wasn't very large but was large enough to work out great. Plus, it had a great wrap-around porch.

When we entered the cabin and I saw that the inside was decorated with trinkets of the Forsters' life. Old license plates and family pictures decorated the log walls.

The main room and the kitchen were not separated by anything and had a small TV that looked like it didn't get used much, and for good reason. A long table was next to the kitchen that was presumably used when the weather wasn't as nice outside. Towards the rear of the house there was a bedroom as well as a bathroom. Upstairs there was a loft with two side by side beds.

We exited the door to the side of the house straight across from where we came in. We walked through the screened in porch and down the stairs to a patio. A fire pit, chairs and outdoor kitchen adorned the patio. While Mr. Forster and I put the motor boat in the lake via boat ramp, Dr. Kuo, Amanda and Rebecca took the canoe out for a spin. We spent much of the afternoon lounging by the lake enjoying the warm spring breeze.

After a while, Dr. and Mrs. Kuo decided they were going to go see the Indian Mounds of the Choctaw Indian tribe. Since I had been in Mississippi, everyone I had talked to had asked if I had seen any of the mounds. I hadn't, but as soon as I told them that, they would say something to the effect of, "Oh well, they're boring. You don't want to see that."

Well, now was my chance. I was here, I might not be again, I was going to see what all the fuss was about with these Indian Mounds. So, I went with Dr. and Mrs. Kuo.

Turns out, everyone was right. They call them "mounds" for a reason. They are literally just hills with grass on them. If I saw it alone, I might not even think anything of it except that it was flat all around it. We climbed up on top and that was about as exciting as it got. The mounds were used for burial purposes, but beyond that, no one can really cite their significance.

By the time we drove back to the cabin, it was almost time for dinner. So we started a fire while Mike Forster started frying up the catfish, French fries and hushpuppies. While he fried, more Forsters showed up and they brought their kids. Then the pastor that hosted the pasta dinner showed up and it was a real, live, Mississippi catfish fry. Inside, Mrs. Forster made coleslaw and tea; both sweet and unsweetened. We all sat around the fire talking, and that's where I learned the origin of hushpuppies.

A long time ago, there was a cook who was frying catfish. His dogs were really annoying him so he took some of the cornmeal, cracked an egg in it, threw some minced onion and other spices, poured in a little buttermilk and made little balls out of the mixture. He deep fried it all and threw it at the dogs saying, "Hush! Puppies!" And they turned out to be delicious.

Dinner was great; and the company was exquisite. All in all, I was very glad I had made a stop in Louisville, Mississippi.

CHAPTER 78

I left Louisville on a Sunday. First, I attended church with the Forsters at the same church that held the dinner two nights prior. I loaded the stroller into Mr. Forster's truck so I could leave right from the church which was across the street from city hall, where I ended three days beforehand. At the conclusion of the service, I met Bubba and Brian outside so I could leave the town with the same people I came into the town with.

When the time came to leave, I said my goodbyes to the Forsters; a family I had become quite attached to and very comfortable around over the past 3 days.

It was disappointing to leave a town where I was a pseudo celebrity, but then again, I was ready to become anonymous again. I was ready to be stared at, honked at, and questioned once again.

Most of all, I was antsy. Two days off had done wonders to my psyche and I thought I would pop if I didn't get to run that day. My thoughts were turned toward the unknown road ahead of me. I was getting close to the end of this journey and only had two more states to cross, one of which was quite thin.

Another person who came out to run with us was a girl by the name of Faith. She was still in high school and competed in Junior Miss Competitions. We each took turns grilling her on what it meant to be a Junior Miss. From what I gathered, Junior Miss is like proving you're a Renaissance man . . . except for high school girls. You have to be good at everything. Her main talent was singing but she said she was also into sports.

Faith was the first one to stop running for the day. She had to get home for a prior commitment. I couldn't blame her, the overcast, humid, and generally gloomy conditions made the day sort of drag on even though the company was great. Bubba and Brian were picked up by Bubba's wife at the county line. Again, I thanked them for coming out and hoped we stayed in touch.

Continuing on by myself was strange. The straight roads and hard pavement were something that I hadn't experienced for two days now, and I believe I had started to forget how to deal with it. This made the end of the day very difficult. I felt like my body had forgotten how to run and my mind had forgotten how to deal with the fact that I still had hundreds of miles to go. I had been completely surrounded by people for the past two and a half days and now I was alone. I used to like being alone for the long days, but now I wasn't so sure of that. Slowly, I convinced myself that once again I would enjoy having all day to occupy my brain with whatever I wanted to occupy it with.

The end of the day brought me to the Miller's house near Macon. Since it was on the exact road I was running on, it was very easy to find. They were very nice people and let me stay in their guest house on a whim because Mr. Forster knew them and put in a good word for me.

CHAPTER 79

The Millers said they had to leave pretty early in the morning but I was welcome to sleep until whenever I wanted, so we said our goodbyes the night before. I appreciated this greatly because I was so tired that night. I was worried that I would be starting over in terms of getting used to the physicality of the run after taking the two days off.

I started to notice a pattern for my off days. I was always more tired the day after I started running again. As long as I kept running and didn't take a day off, I was fine.

I woke up the next morning at 7 am feeling well rested and ready to go, so I started. The road I was on turned a hard left at one point and joined up with a road that went straight north for about a half of a mile, then split right to head east once again.

On that northbound road I crossed a small bridge entering the town of Macon. While I was on the bridge, a truck pulled into the parking lot ahead of me. He waited there until I got a little closer and he rolled down his window.

"Hey I saw you on TV!"

"Yep, that was me in Louisville."

He asked if he could take my picture and I agreed that it would be fine. He and his son had just finished hunting, so they were dressed all in hunting camouflage. They got out and went to the back of it. He then pulled out a huge dead turkey by the feet and dropped it on the ground! I was instantly stoked. I'd seen pictures of hunters with their turkeys, but I had never seen one fresh off the kill. I crouched down next to it just like I had seen other hunters do, and got my picture taken.

This was also the day I crossed into Alabama. The weather was fantastic and there wasn't a single cloud in the sky. Farmland seemed to roll on forever but unlike the ranches in Texas, this farmland was mostly green and most had tractors rolling over it getting the soil ready for planting.

I ran into Aliceville, Alabama through the west side. I learned later that this was not the greatest part of town, though I had no trouble here.

The first gas station in town called my name and welcomed me inside. An icy cold Coca Cola Classic was on the menu and I couldn't pass it up. Walking down the street through the beginning of town while sipping on my refreshing beverage, I passed a house with more people on the porch than a fire marshal would probably be happy with. Everyone looked at me funny while I walked on the sidewalk in front of their house. One person shouted at me,

"Hey! What are you doing? Is there a baby in there?"

"Nope, it's all my stuff!"

"Where you goin?

"The Atlantic Ocean."

"Sweet Jesus! Where did you come from?"

"The Pacific Ocean."

"You came here, from the Pacific Ocean on foot? Where's that? California?"

"Yep, I'm running across the country."

"Damn boy, you skinny enough for it."

They all just about lost their minds laughing at that one. I laughed too. They told me to be safe and stay out of that part of town at night. "Specially 'cause of my white skin." I thanked them for the advice and waved goodbye.

I had to meet up with Mrs. Lavender. I was a bit early, but I thought it would be alright.

When I ran to the intersection where I was to meet Mrs. Lavender, she was already there waiting with a newspaper reporter. Mrs. Lavender was about 5 foot 5 inches with blonde hair, and a petite build. She had a large smile on her face and giant sun glasses. I had no idea how old she was, but she was very welcoming and had a great southern accent. She was standing there with a peanut butter sandwich, a banana and water.

The reporter asked me some questions, and then parted ways. Right where I ended happened to be in front of the Aliceville Museum. Mrs. Lavender suggested we go in and take a quick look around because it's what Aliceville was famous for.

During World War II Aliceville was home to a giant prisoner of war camp. The camp had capacity for 6,000 prisoners and employed 1,000 people to run the camp. Though it was a prison camp, the biggest surprise to me was how well everyone was treated. The Geneva Convention was followed very strictly. Prisoners and guards actually became friends. They show a documentary in the museum and it revealed that Aliceville had a big celebration called the Friendship Reunion in 1989 and again in 1993 where some of the German prisoners came back with their families to visit with old friends they made with the guards at this camp.

I was surprised that stories like this were not shared more often. This was a situation where people could have been beaten, treated unjustly, and made miserable. Instead they were treated with respect and in a justified, humane manner. Yet, this is not the story we heard on the news or in our history books at school. We only heard about the POW camps that starved people and beat them without mercy. True friendships evolved from what could have been a terrible encounter for both sides of the camp.

Afterwards, Mrs. Lavender brought me out to their cabin where we met up with Mr. Lavender. Mr. Lavender and I rode his big Gator (which is sort of like a golf cart on steroids) around his land and showed me where he hunts.

Being out in the woods was nice. I missed the trees and being on trails. He had several little huts built where he could sit and wait for deer to come into the field.

At dinner that night, several people came over for dinner; including the people I was planning to stay with the following night. The company was great and it was nice to get a preview of the people I was staying with tomorrow.

CHAPTER 80

Eutaw was a tiny little town; quaint and cozy. Running there was interesting because the roads were smaller and there was far less traffic, which I always welcomed.

When I arrived at the town, I was very hungry. I saw a man walking toward me on the sidewalk. I stopped him and asked him where a good local place to grab a bite to eat was. He pointed me two doors down from where I was to a barbeque place called, Truman's. I met up with Mr. Eatman afterward and he drove me back to their house. They lived about 45 minutes from where I stopped, so I greatly appreciated the effort they made to drive all that way to come pick me up.

The drive to their house was all on back roads and was a welcomed change.

Arriving at their house, I was taken aback. The house had belonged to Mr. Eatman's parents and had been built in the late 1800s. Plantation style with lots of land around and a big barn that he used as storage, the house was beautifully kept and magnificent to say the least. As we drove around back to where the garage was, I saw smoke coming from the far side of the patio. When I got out, I knew exactly what it was.

Mr. Eatman was a turkey hunter, and this was his freshest kill. Saying that Mr. Eatman is a mere turkey hunter is a gross understatement. During turkey hunting season, which is March 15 to April 30, he goes every morning without fail.

After getting cleaned up, I visited with Mr. and Mrs. Eatman. He told me that he was a timber farmer. He asked if I wanted to see his land, and I couldn't turn it down. We climbed in his golf cart on steroids and started off down the trail with his two dogs running as fast as they could down the trail ahead of us.

I really wanted to get out of the cart and run with the dogs. It had been forever since I ran on a trail. I was very envious of those dogs. They would be running down the trail and then would run around a curve in the trail. Next time we saw them they'd be chasing a squirrel somewhere off the trail. When they stopped, they would pant for a minute just looking at us with those giant dog-smiles on their faces. They were in their element, and they were in my element, too.

Mr. Eatman explained how the timber business worked. I was very curious because you always hear about the tree hugging hippies complaining about cutting trees, but you never get to hear the timber farmer's point of view.

He explained it to me like this: The forest naturally goes through phases. Trees are planted, they grow, after many years, they die, fall, and rot . . . just like humans. Timber farmers don't cut all their trees at once. They cut them a few acres at a time so while one plot is being cut, the other plots are in different stages of their life cycle. This way, there are always new trees being planted, and there are always trees living, and there are usually trees ready to be cut and sold. Also, most of his trees were on an 80 year cycle so timber farming is usually a family business.

He loved his land. I could tell that he enjoyed being out there, driving around his land scouting how certain plots were coming along and seeing what kind of work needed to be done. Some of the trails had freshly fallen trees and the cart had no problem traversing these obstacles. We were bounced around the cab of the cart and it made the ride slightly like a roller coaster.

At one point we hit a rather large bump in the trail and it caused me to fly forward and whack my knee on the front of the cart where a dashboard would be had it been a car. It hurt so badly. It conveniently hit right where the sharp pain still existed from the day back in Texas that forced me to walk all day. The spot was still tender to the touch but was very manageable during running. I think Mr. Eatman felt worse than my knee did even though it wasn't his fault. Sure enough, after much rubbing, it felt fine once again.

After driving around on the intricate system of trails that divided his acres of land, we made our way back to the house. Being out on the trails was incredibly relaxing and gave me a huge boost in energy. It was like my nature battery was somewhat charged and I was able to look at the days ahead of me with some anticipation as I looked forward to reaching the end and returned to running on trails.

Upon retuning to the house, we all relaxed and visited with some guests they had for dinner. The fresh turkey was incredible and I had no idea it would be so different from the store bought turkey. It was slightly wilder tasting, but don't let that sound like a bad thing.

The meat was juicy and fresh, and since it was slowly smoked over the course of the day, it was cooked to perfection. Mr. Eatman had opened my eyes to the reason so many people were big into turkey hunting around Alabama.

The following morning Mrs. Eatman drove me back to my stopping point in Eutaw and I thanked her and we said our goodbyes.

CHAPTER 81

The next day was sunny in the mid 70s without a cloud in sight. A great day for running. I got several ride offers. Today, unlike when it was raining or snowing, it was much easier to turn the offers down.

When I got into Greensboro, I walked through the town and there it was; Pie Lab. A shop dedicated to nothing more than pies. Whether I wanted to or not, I had to try it. It was beyond my control.

My first slice was pear and blackberry. Heavenly. It was so tasty; warm and comforting. The fruit in it was just right; not too crunchy, and not too soft. The crust: flakey and buttery but not too salty. I knew that the pies in this place were well thought out and had much work put into them. I had to try another. One kind of pie was calling my name; peanut butter, honey and banana. I said to myself, "That pie will be mine."

I made it mine. This one had the ratio of perfection. Every ingredient was carefully placed in the mixture and contributed equally to my thorough enjoyment of this pie eating experience. Feeling comfortably full of pie and incredibly satisfied I bought another slice to save for later. I left the contemporary-looking shop where many people were working on laptops sipping coffee and enjoying slices of pie.

CHAPTER 82

Sometimes paths cross for specific reasons. We don't know why at the time, but we meet again later on down the road. The following day, as I was running into the town of Marion, this came into play. My dad, who had been helping me this whole time by looking ahead at the towns I was going through for places and connections where I could stay, looked in Marion for a place for me to stay just like always. This time, he found something that would be very helpful and was an incredible coincidence.

My dad had been in the Marine Corps for 20 years; most of that time was spent as a helicopter pilot. The friendships he made during this period had lasted a lifetime.

As my dad was scanning the town over the internet from our home in Stafford, VA, he came across Marion Military Institute. His immediate thoughts turned toward his own military connections and the unspoken bond of taking care of each other and each others' families'. He went to the website for the institute and looked at the home page for contact information. As he scanned the page, a familiar face jumped out at him. MMI's president, Col. David Mollahan looked very familiar and he instantly remembered that this man was in my dad's first squadron back in southern California.

He contacted him, and Col. Mollahan had no problem with me staying with him where he and his wife lived at the institute.

I ran into town and took a right to head toward the institute. It was conveniently where I needed to turn to stay on my route. The town was quaint, and warm, though there weren't many people. The people I did see were nice and everyone waved to me. At least, that's how I took it; maybe they were waving AT me to get out of the town or were signaling danger to me. Either way, they did so with a smile on their face.

Approaching the institute I saw the giant sign just inside the gate leading to the grounds. On the marquee, along with several other cycling announcements was a quote from Lance Armstrong, "Pain is temporary, but quitting is forever." I found this a bit ironic. Had I been thinking about quitting, I definitely would've thought twice about it after seeing that.

On the main lawn, I saw many students all dressed in various physical training uniforms performing different tasks. Some groups were doing push-ups, some were doing jumping jacks, and still others were practicing their drill routine with their rifles. None of them were standing around with nothing to do. I found this most impressive for a school. Everyone was moving and seemed determined to get somewhere.

As I walked up the main street of the institute, I saw a smiling woman who I could only guess recognized me and was looking for me.

Ingrid was Col Mollahan's wife and was incredibly cheery. When I first met her she said I looked like a McGlade and told me how much I looked like my dad. It was even more ironic because back when she knew my dad, he was only a couple years older than I was now. It must have been a little bit like a time warp seeing me now.

She gave me a tour of the campus and then a tour of the house. The house they live in is the President of the Institute's house. The rooms on the bottom floor are reserved mostly for hosting important people. Parlors, and tea rooms, and a living room that looked like it belonged in the White House. It was all very impressive. The upstairs was for living. That is where most of the bedrooms were, and also a more relaxed living room with an entertainment system.

After cleaning up, a reporter from the campus newspaper came by the house for an interview. The normal questions were answered, but the feel was very informal. Mrs. Mollahan stuck around because I think she had a few questions of her own. Before too long, Col. Mollahan came home and I was finally able to meet this old friend of my dad's.

For dinner that night we went to a pot luck dinner at the Officer's Club. They call it Dinner Club and it is a monthly pot luck dinner. Most of the people that came out were at least 65 with a few outliers in their 50s but everyone was incredibly welcoming. Mostly retired military families, they asked me questions about the run, and I was happy to answer their questions. They were a quirky bunch and completed the age range that I hadn't talked to yet. I had talked to little kids, high school kids, kids my own age, young families, middle aged families, and now I had completed the ages. There was even a couple in their nineties.

I have always enjoyed eating. Not to say I'm a glutton or anything, or even that I have "expensive taste buds," I just enjoy good food. Especially home cooked food, because everyone has their own little twist on recipes. It is this reason that I love pot lucks. Everyone brings their own side dish, usually home cooked, you lay it on a table and everyone goes at it. It is a genius idea. There is also something about running across a country that makes people want to feed you. As soon as people learn you are exerting a certain amount of energy for several hours a day, they want to give you food.

Mixing my love for food, my love for pot lucks, and everyone else's desire to feed me made this event even more pleasant than just being in the presence of good company. They were nice people who were genuinely interested in what I was doing. The evening was a great experience, and I can comfortably say I made some new friends.

CHAPTER 83

Waking up the next morning, I started running early because I was meeting my Aunt Marie, someone I have known since I was a couple weeks old. The Mollahans walked me out to the gate of the campus and took my picture next to the Lance Armstrong quote. I thanked them again, and took off in the early morning mist. If the air was still, the temperature felt higher because of the humidity. If a breeze kicked up, the air felt cooler against my skin.

It wasn't long before I was out of the town and solely on the back roads that would take me to Selma, Alabama. Traffic was scarce, and as the sun rose higher off the horizon, the shadows became shorter and the temperature rose quickly. Though it never got too hot, I was trying to run faster than I normally would because I wanted to get to Selma before my aunt did. She was driving south from Huntsville and was meeting me in Selma to take me back to her house so I could take a couple of days off for Easter and spend time with my Uncle Rich, Aunt Marie and cousins, Chris and Mia.

When I was about 10 miles outside of Selma I received a call from Marie saying she would be driving on the road I was running on so I could put the stroller in her van and not have to push it through town.

With about 8 miles to go, she met up with me. I was able to get rid of the stroller even if it was just for 8 miles.

"Hey! It's the emaciated running man!" She said as she climbed out of the Toyota van.

"Whoa whoa, watch who you're calling emaciated."

"Actually, no, you're not emaciated at all, you look surprisingly good."

"Thanks, it's good to see you too."

We planned that she would drive up the road for a couple miles and meet me and leap frog until I was done for the day. As soon as I turned around to run the remaining 8 miles something inside of me snapped. I felt wild and very free. Somewhat shackled by the jogger, I no longer needed to lug that thing down the road dodging cars, playing 'chicken' with them, and hoping they would turn. I could run on the soft shoulder in the dirt and almost feel like I was on a trail again.

This wildness flowed through my blood and pumped the blood through my legs. They churned quickly and I floated down the road lightly and like a bullet. I was going so much faster than I had been and it was unbelievably freeing.

It was a slight concern of mine that after this whole ordeal I wasn't going to be able to run fast anymore. I thought, and had heard that running long and slow everyday would make me slower and after this it would be a very large task to learn how to move my legs quicker again. Though, in hindsight, this is all true; right then, I was sure it was false. Light on my feet, I was running fast.

After turning left to take the route to the north side of town so that I wouldn't have to go through downtown and deal with even more traffic, I was now running around all the normal outskirt-of-town-businesses. Fast food chains, new and used car dealerships, pawn shops and more shopping centers than I could count, it was a generally unpleasant place to run. Up ahead, on my left, I saw a group of people standing in a Wendy's parking lot. I tried not to think anything of it, and actually tried not to look at them because nothing says awkward like staring back at a group of people who is staring at you while you're running through a town with shorter-than-average-shorts. Besides, I was listening to the band Converge on repeat for the 90th time that day and my thought process couldn't be interrupted.

As I passed the entrance to the parking lot where the family was standing I casually glanced over just to make sure they weren't signaling me and actually were just staring. But when I looked at them, I recognized them. It was the JP and his family who I had stayed with the previous week and had floated the river with. Shocked, I stopped to talk to them. They were on their way to their grandma's house for Easter and had seen me running down the road and decided it would be a good time to stop for lunch. Seeing them was a nice little boost and put a great ending on a potentially very awkward stare-down session.

Upon reaching the end of town, I climbed into the minivan and Aunt Marie and I started down the road on our way to Huntsville, Alabama. She's a great person to road trip with, and this was very important because we had a three and a half hour drive ahead of us; which also meant she had just driven three and a half hours to come pick me up.

Upon arriving in Huntsville, I was greeted by my Uncle Rich and my cousins Chris and Mia. Being around family was very relaxing. I enjoyed meeting new people and staying in towns I had never been to, but even though I had never been to this house of theirs (my uncle was in the Army so they moved around a great deal), just being around them felt more like home.

CHAPTER 84

The next couple days were spent relaxing with my mom's brother and his family in Huntsville, Alabama. The NASA space camp is in Huntsville so we visited that, and visited Mia's horse, Max.

We also spent our time playing with their dog, Ginger, which is a Portuguese water dog and is incredibly smart. She can do some crazy tricks. One that my aunt showed me was she looked at Ginger, made her hand into a little gun and said, "Bang!" Ginger dropped to the floor with her head still up. Marie said, "Bang!" one more time and Ginger put her head on the ground and stayed there until we worshipped her for completing the trick.

Easter came, and we went to their church which was huge. That afternoon, I packed up and Aunt Marie and I left for Selma, the last town I had run to. The drive back was just as pleasant as the drive up to the house. This time though, I was dropped where I stopped and I ran for about an hour or two just to see how far I got in that time. Then, Marie picked me up and we went to a little house that someone in the area had donated to us for the night. It felt strange to leave and I dreaded it a little. Being here was like being at home, and now that I was home, I felt a little like I was done, and didn't need to keep running.

Unfortunately, I was brought back to reality the next morning and continued running.

CHAPTER 85

We left the little house very early so I could start running. The Arthritis Foundation of Alabama had a lot planned for me that day and I needed to finish early.

Starting out was gloomy. The air was thick with fog and I couldn't see more than 100 yards ahead of me. I ran with my headlamp even though it was daylight because I thought it might be safer. The ground was wet and made the tires produce a constant buzzing sort of sound. On these back roads there were minimal cars which I was pleased with and added to the serenity of the early morning. Even though the air was cool in the low to mid 50's, it was very humid. I became drenched in sweat quickly. The fog added to the scenery, as ironic as that sounds. The forest surrounding the road was thick, lush and green. Having shapes in front of me be mere blobs and then take shape as they emerged from the fog gave my surroundings a still and mysterious life of they own. The quietness was amplified by the cloud that hovered only inches from the ground and dampened not only the street but also any sound that tried to reach my ears.

Before too long, the fog began to lift, the day warmed up and the sun came out. I continued to run without walking breaks because I didn't want to be late. I was meeting the Crowes, a family who had a child with Arthritis and was going to be taking me several places throughout the day. I talked to them and they gave me some directions to the YMCA where I was to meet them. Mrs. Crowe said, "When you see the giant hill, you're almost there."

Sure enough, from around a corner, appeared a hill with no top. Cars just seemed to keep driving up.

Of course this is at the very end of the day, I sarcastically said to myself. Sometimes, when there's nothing else to do, you just have to put your head down, and make things just a little harder for yourself. So I decided to run the hill just to get it over with.

I met the Crowes at the Rite Aid at the top of the hill and I loaded my stroller into their van. They drove me to the YMCA so I could shower before they brought me to the school to talk to the kids. When I was finished in the shower and came back out, the owner of the YMCA was waiting for me at the front desk. I thanked him for letting me use his facilities complimentary. He responded with a donation.

After snapping a few pictures, we got back in the van and headed to Pine Level Elementary School.

Upon reaching the school, I met a few of the teachers and they brought me to a classroom with only one child coloring a picture at one of the tables in the room. I was a bit confused about where all the kids were until the principal came and told me I'd be speaking to the whole school in the cafeteria.

After a minute or two they came back and brought me to the cafeteria. I was very surprised that there were about 450 kids. It was just a sea of kids all sitting cross-legged on the floor of the giant room. To the left of the door where I entered was a stage with a pull-down screen where a projector was displaying many of the pictures I had taken and had posted on my Facebook page and blog.

I was not expecting the amount of kids or the stage or the picture projector. I'm not sure what I was expecting but that wasn't it. The principal climbed the three steps to the stage and took the microphone off of the stand. She quieted the kids with an authority I hadn't heard since I was in elementary school.

She did it in the least abrasive way possible.

"Alright everyone, we have a special guest today . . ." She said in a soft voice.

In those eight words it got so quiet, you could have heard a mouse fart if there had been a mouse that had gotten a hold of some of the beans that were served in the cafeteria that day.

" . . . his name is Patrick McGlade and he is running across the country for kids with Arthritis. So here is Patrick." The kids clapped and the principal gave me the microphone. The kids sat there patiently waiting for me to start telling them why I would choose to take on the task of running across the country. The teachers lined the sides of the mass of kids like prison guards except, thankfully, none of them were holding rifles or beating sticks. I had spoken to many schools at this point in the trip, yet, until I started talking, this one was the most intimidating. I gave them the "who, what, when, where, and how" and then asked them if they had any questions, just like I did with every school I had talked to. Every kid seemed to have a question. It was hard to choose but usually I just picked out a random kid's shirt color and answered their question. Most of the questions were very similar to the questions that other kids from other schools asked.

After sharing stories with the kids and answering questions for about 20 minutes. The principal gave me the 3 more questions signal. In case you were curious about what that looks like, it is where you, the person calling the shots, raises your hand and waves it a little bit, and then you hold up three fingers and mouth, "Three more." Even with the last three questions, there were still dozens of kids with their hands in the air. I felt kind of bad not being able to answer everyone's questions but it was time for them to go home.

Following the school, the Crowes drove me to city hall where the mayor declared it "Patrick McGlade Day." He said since it was technically *my day*, I could rob a bank and cause some sort of ruckus throughout the town and not get in trouble for it . . . until tomorrow.

Following our rendezvous with the mayor, I did a quick interview with a reporter. Then, the Crowes and I walked through the town and went into a little shop to get some ice cream. While making my decision, I was informed that even though the white board told me they had rocky road, they were out. That's when I realized that this was going to be a problem, but then again, it is ice cream, and every flavor is delicious . . . except cotton candy.

To finish off the day, the Crowes, the Alabama Arthritis Foundation, a couple of families with kids with arthritis and I went to Ryan's Restaurant for dinner. We all sat at a long table and talked the evening away. It was there that I met a little girl named Meredith. She is a very well spoken and outgoing 9 year old with arthritis. She has been a spokesperson for juvenile arthritis for many walks and other arthritis events. It was nice to meet her because I would be with her on the news for an interview the next day.

That night I went home with Mr. and Mrs. Hemphill, where I would stay for the next 3 nights. Mrs. Hemphill was very involved with the Arthritis Foundation and was incredible with helping me raise JA awareness over the next couple days. They were an interesting couple. They were a middle aged couple who had kids that were already grown. After spending a couple of days with them I realized they were one of those couples that genuinely enjoy being around each other, yet, not in a gross-me-out kind of way.

CHAPTER 86

April 6th probably would have been easier as a day off. I had so much going on that day I had to split up the run into two parts. The morning was an early start so I could run as far as I could before I was picked up by Mrs. Hemphill and brought to the first engagement.

The upside of staying in the same place is that I didn't have to push the jogger for two days. The upside of that is that I can run faster without the jogger. Right from the start, I booked it. As I continued down the road in Alabama, I noticed the increase in humidity and tried to get as far as I could before the heat kicked in. Luckily, since I had to be finished with the first part of the run by 10 am, I would be busy with activities during the hottest part of the day.

Like clockwork, Mrs. Hemphill rolled up in her car next to me at 9:59 and had some refreshments for me waiting in a cooler in the car. I was able to squeeze in 17 miles and got through downtown Montgomery, AL, which only left 10 for the evening. The first stop Mrs. Hemphill had planned for me was to go see a friend of hers at the baseball stadium in Montgomery. I was very excited to go by the stadium for several reasons. The first was I really enjoy going to baseball games and like seeing different stadiums. Even though the official season didn't start until the following week, I still wanted to see the stadium. The second reason I was stoked was the team name. Montgomery, Alabama's baseball team name is The Biscuits . . . like the fluffy pastry. Need I say more?

When we stopped over there, we looked around the brand spanking new stadium and I wished that the first game was tonight rather than next week. I was able to meet one of the team managers and she let me pick out a shirt. I was very appreciative and picked one that had the mascot on it which, of course, is a biscuit smiling with a pad of butter as the tongue. After thanking her again, we departed the stadium for the NBC studio for an interview.

Mrs. Hemphill and I met Meredith and her mom over at the studio and we decided it would be best for Meredith to join me in the same interview instead of doing two separate interviews. I was just fine with that because that meant that the information on arthritis was coming from someone actually afflicted and so it would be much more accurate, and mean that much more.

Even more than the night before, her well spoken nature and intelligence shone through her 9 year old little body. While you're talking to her, you would never guess that she actually has it until she starts listing off the intense medications she is on. During the interview I was very happy to share the stage, or couch as the case was, with her because she was clearly more comfortable in front of the giant cameras and lights and in turn, her confidence helped ease some of my nerves. She was so comfortable that I wouldn't be surprised if someday she has her own talk show.

After thanking the news station, and saying goodbye to Meredith and her mother, Mrs. Hemphill and I departed the station and made our way down town to grab some lunch between engagements and sight seeing. For lunch, we went to Chris' Hotdogs. The local eatery has been around since 1917 and has served some very famous people as the pictures on the wall will remind you. The dogs came fully slathered in slaw, cabbage, or sauerkraut. I couldn't decide exactly what else was on it but it also had a killer sauce on top. Because of the amount of condiments and toppings, toward the end, a spoon may have been helpful. As gross as it sounds, it was delicious and I can see why it has been there for close to 93 years.

Next—the sights. We were close to the capitol so we went to see that, and took a quick look inside. After deciding that quantity was more important than quality, we only stayed for about 5 minutes. Just long enough to walk around the inside and look at the paintings of former governors. From there we went to the Civil Rights Museum and the Rosa Parks museum but didn't actually go inside either. We also went to the church where Martin Luther King preached. Unfortunately the doors were locked so we were not able to go into that one. It had occurred to me that the Civil Rights March of 1965 had gone from Selma, AL to Montgomery, AL and much of my route was very similar to the route they had taken. It was a lot to think about that part of my journey was a route that so many people had also taken fighting for their rights as equals. I was very happy I had chosen to travel the southern half of the country because

I was able to travel a piece of history on foot the same way Dr. Martin Luther King had.

After seeing all these sights, it was time to go to city hall where we met the mayor of Montgomery's assistant. Following the meeting were two radio interviews. The last interview was for a public radio station through a local college and was by far the most in depth interview I had ever done. They were the questions that I hadn't thought about before she asked. Things like what I thought about when I was alone for so many hours per day, how good my contact was with my family and friends, how I started running, and what benefits it provided me as far as physical health and other aspects of my life. She asked about feelings and quite frankly, it made me a bit uncomfortable to answer questions like that to someone I had just met and over a radio station that was being pumped out over the airwaves to several of the surrounding counties. My in-depth answers were going to be heard by people who didn't know me, and who I would never get to meet. It was a bit strange to say the least.

After so much talking, and meeting so many people, I was wiped out. It was time to recharge my battery and go for a run. Luckily, I had some more miles I had to catch up on. Since I had been busy all day, it was now 3:30 and the heat had risen throughout the day. I started where I had left off, as usual, and at 92 degrees, it was the hottest day I had run in so far.

CHAPTER 87

The following morning brought with it more activities in the form of a breakfast with the team leaders for the Arthritis Foundation's walk in Alabama. I was able to talk to them about what I was doing and the importance of fundraising for the event. Since it was a group of adults, I didn't get the normal questions about how I relieved myself while running or anything like that.

From the breakfast, Mr. Hemphill drove me to the starting point of the day's run and I began my day. The temperature was cooler than the previous day but it was 97% humidity so it didn't take long to feel warmer than it was.

Due to a healthy dose of pancakes that morning, I was well energized and before too long, I arrived in Tuskegee. Mrs. Hemphill met me to take me back to their house where I would be spending my last night with them. Before we left Tuskegee, we visited the memorial to the Tuskegee Airmen, the first black military airmen during World War II.

After returning to the Montgomery area, we met up with congressman Mike Rogers and were able to talk to him about arthritis. That night we had salmon with a brown sugar and soy sauce mixture and it was incredible.

CHAPTER 88

Leaving Tuskegee with my jogger felt like an undertaking. When I woke up the morning of April 8th it was raining. My immediate thoughts were negative but I had to get down the road anyway. It rained on the whole drive out to Tuskegee but as soon as we reached the parking lot where I had ended in, it stopped raining. I thanked Mr. Hemphill for all his help and for providing me with a place to stay for the past three days.

Of course, as soon as I stepped out of the car, it started raining again. Starting to run down the road and through the town, thunder rolled and the rain fell lightly on my head and stroller covered in the water-proof cover that I had brought.

Not three miles down the road, my feet were already soaking wet and my clothes hung on me like they were a few sizes too big. The rain gradually fell heavier throughout the day. Luckily it was warm outside.

During a particularly straight section of road, I was running up a hill while a river of ankle deep water was going the opposite way and was covering my feet. Between coming up for air, the 6 foot high waves that trucks tossed my way, and the large caliber bullet-sized drops that so graciously allowed my view to not exceed 20 feet in front of the jogger, I started laughing.

Soaked to the bone, pushing a baby jogger, dodging semi trucks and in desperate need of scuba gear, it just seemed funny to me at the time. Maybe I had lost it.

About a mile from the intersection that was Marvyn, it stopped raining and I was able to call Kenton. The nephew of JP Watson, who I had stayed with in

Mississippi, went to Auburn University and I was directly south of Auburn by about 40 minutes. He met me at the intersection and he gave me a ride to the hotel that was donated that night. And after dropping me off at the hotel to take a shower that wasn't exactly needed due to the amount of water that I had already encountered, he showed me around Auburn University which is, as it turns out, a very nice campus with a gigantic football stadium.

The following morning, Kenton picked me up and brought me back to Marvyn, and after thanking him for all of his help, I started running toward Georgia.

CHAPTER 89

The day I ran into Georgia felt like entering the last mile of a race, or walking into the class that you would take your last final for the year. I didn't have much to go, it would be mostly flat, and I was still so busy with answering emails, and keeping up with who I was meeting and where, I didn't have a whole lot of time to think about things other than the finish.

That running day took forever. Time just seems to move slower when you're anticipating a big city like Columbus to spring out of the ground.

Before I reached Columbus, though, the road took a drastic turn for the worst. The shoulder disappeared and high speed traffic picked up without warning. It was a mess and it took forever to get down the road. My time on the road consisted of sprinting from one driveway or side road to another in between breaks in heavy traffic, or diving off the road and pulling my jogger with me when I wouldn't make it in time.

After I seemed to get the hang of the sprinting routine down, a news reporter called me and asked if we could meet up and do an interview. I had no problem with this, but didn't think that my stop and go running style would be ideal for him, but he didn't sound too concerned on the phone.

We met up and the semi-stout, gray haired man's first comments were about how terrible the traffic was for getting "the right shot," but we did the interview quickly anyway. I was kind of surprised at how much of the interview process I had learned from all the other interviews I had done so far. He asked me my name and what I was doing, and I went through my whole list answering the "who, what, when, where, how, how to donate and why" questions. When I stopped at the end he just sort of looked at me like,

"Geeze, kid, you read my mind."

He only asked me if there was anything else I wanted to add, and since I had already gone through it all, I declined the offer to keep speaking.

As he lowered his camera, he asked, "So, you do a lot of these huh?" I had to reply with a simple, "Yes."

I reassured myself I was not going the wrong way by asking him how far Columbus was from where we were and he told me it was just about three miles away. I apologized for being in such a hurry to leave, but I had waited 3 months to see the welcome to Georgia sign, and I was anxious. He said he completely understood; I was on my way once again.

The sprinting routine continued until I entered the outskirts of Columbus and then the sidewalks started. I wasn't particularly fond of the sidewalks and the way they would dip down and pop up suddenly to accommodate driveways, but it sure beat the alternative of getting hit by a car. After what seemed like an eternity, many turns, and thinking I might have been lost a few times, I saw the bridge that took me into Columbus, GA. I saw the sign that said, "Welcome to Georgia." I was both unimpressed and extremely relieved to see it at the same time. The other signs for entering states had been huge monstrosities, often with the state theme and slogan, as well as the state flag painted on them. This one was a plain square about 3 ft x 3 ft. Black, block letters on a green square sign. I had waited so long to see it I didn't even care that it didn't personally welcome me into the state of Georgia. It might as well have said, "Welcome home Patrick! We've been expecting you." Also there by the sign was the reporter. He was standing there, camera ready and so I waved to him as I started running over the bridge into Georgia.

Running through downtown cities has never been the ideal running place for me but this experience was a little different. Columbus was a nice city, and I seemed to hit every part of the city as I made my way through it on my way to the hotel where I was scheduled to stay. The nice parts were very nice, and the not so nice parts were a complete 180.

Crossing one bridge there was a homeless man sitting at the foot of the bridge wearing several sweaters and a winter coat along with long sweat pants. He was surrounded by boxes and trash and a shopping cart. It wasn't garbage in the sense that it was just old "junk" that no one would want. It was trash like old wrappers, crumbled paper, and garbage bags with holes in them containing banana peels, other rotting food. The stench as I ran by was horrific and the wave of rotting food, hot trash, and excruciatingly severe body odor rushed my nostrils and all pre-thoughts about stopping and talking with the man went straight out the window because I was afraid I might barf. He wasn't the first homeless person I saw asleep on the sidewalk in the mid-day's heat; nor was he the last; but something stuck with me after seeing him.

While I wandered the streets of Columbus, I thought about what happened to put him in this situation, and if there was anything that could be done to help him. Then I thought about my reasoning for not stopping to help him. Was the smell that bad? Was helping him not worth waking him up? While I didn't know what I could have even done to help him, I couldn't find answers to these questions, and that disappointed me.

When I finally found my hotel I went to the check in desk and they had a box for me. I was somewhat surprised because usually, if my parents sent it, they told me so that I was sure not to forget to ask about it. When I read the return address, it wasn't from them at all. It was a Georgia address and I didn't recognize the name right away. I maneuvered my rig around the halls to my room with the package tucked under my arm like a football thinking where I had heard the name before. As soon as I got into the room, I tore into the package and it occurred to me exactly where I had heard the name before. It was the Arthritis Foundation of Georgia who had sent the package as a "Welcome to our state" package. It was great! There was a very nice note from them, peanuts, because that's what they grow in Georgia, and a blanket in there along with other little foodstuffs and goodies. It was very nice of them to surprise me with the package. The peanuts were delicious and I immediately indulged in the tasty legume.

I had gotten a call earlier in the day from a man who was involved with the Columbus Running Club who had invited me for dinner. I didn't know him ahead of time but if someone is offering me dinner, there is a good chance I won't decline the offer.

John picked me up and drove me to his house which was just north of Columbus in some great looking back country where he told me about all these trails that he had built on his land. John was an ultra runner as well, so we talked about everything ultra runners talk about. Turns out, he was a rather serious ultra runner. He had completed the "Grand Slam of Ultra running." This consists of finishing the Western States 100 Mile Endurance Run, Vermont 100 Mile Endurance Run, Leadville Trail 100 Mile Run and the Wasatch Front 100

Mile Endurance Run all in the same year. He also does a run across Georgia called the Run for the Heroes. But, instead of doing it in 11 days, with an extra day off in between like I was going to be doing, he did it in 4 days the past two years. In 2010, he did it in 3. Serious runner.

His house was beautiful. He built it himself out of logs and he owned his own construction business, so he really knew what he was doing. We had dinner with his wife, Melissa, his daughter, Emma and his friend Troy and his family came over as well. The three guys who had run a similar route across the country before me had stayed with John. It was cool to meet both of them and put faces to the names that the three guys had told me about.

During dinner, John asked me what I had planned for the next day. It was a scheduled day off, and I had no plans at all.

"Well, some of the guys and girls from the running club are getting together to a little run tomorrow. Are you interested?" he asked?

"What kind of run?"

"It's called the beer mile."

"What time?"

"7:00"

"I'm there."

Turns out, the Columbia Underground Running Club had a race that is growing in popularity throughout the U.S. It's called the Beer Mile. Of course it's a race, so the objective is to win, but it's not just a running race; there is beer involved, so not throwing up is also the goal.

The race takes place on a quarter mile track, or an out-and-back course. When the starter says, "On your marks, get set, chug!" you pick up your first can of beer and chug it. Then you run a quarter mile. When you reach the starting line again, you chug another beer, then run your second quarter mile. Repeat the cycle for the third quarter mile and the fourth. When all is said and done, one mile is run and 4 cans of beer are consumed. This is how it was explained to me the night before the big race.

That night, John let me borrow his truck to drive back to the hotel. He also said I could use it the next day if I wanted to tour the city a little faster than on foot. I thought he was nuts. Here is some stranger that he just met a few hours ago and he gave me his truck to drive around in while I was in the area. I was semi in shock, but then it occurred to me, "This is just a ploy to make sure I show up for the Beer Mile."

CHAPTER 90

When I met up with John the next afternoon, he was doing some repairs on the house. These were no ordinary chores. The guy was replacing a whole bathroom on the third floor. He was doing this of course after he had woken up at 3:00 am and gone for a 20 or so mile run.

We went down to his business workshop and put the finishing touches on the trophies for the race. A 4x4x12 block of stained and finished wood with beer bottle caps riveted to the top. An old track shoe spray painted gold was screwed to the top and was the prize to be given to the top male and top female winners. There must have been at least 40 bottle caps on each block of wood. He must have either had the idea a few months back and started collecting the caps then, or had one crazy night of "work" collecting the caps. He had planned for it to be a yearly prize so that whoever won this year would have to come back next year to retain, or lose, the prized trophy. When it was all done, it was a work of art; such craftsmanship went into the formation of the sheer beauty that sat before my eyes.

John, his wife and I piled into her Mini Cooper and drove out to his friend's house where the mile long race would take place. When we arrived, there was already a crowd present and the course was marked out in cones. A straight line course: out and back would equal a quarter mile. We signed up, and received our bib numbers, our shirts and chose our elixirs. Before long, they were explaining the rules and we got ready.

"On your marks . . . . get set . . . . CHUG!"

We were off! . . . sort of. We each cracked our first beer and began chugging. It was very cold and went down like ice. But soon enough I began running. I was in third place after the first chug but caught second place on the way out. On the way back for the first quarter mile I caught the first place guy and moved into first place. I hadn't run *just* a mile for time since I was in high school, and back then, I wasn't in the best shape. I opened my second beer, held my breath, and chugged. Then a guy coming back from his first lap threw up looking much like the scene from The Exorcist. It would be a tough race. I took one breath in between the whole second can and then started running again, still in first place. Half mile down, and still in first place I opened my third beer and chugged. Third lap down and on my last beer I knew it'd be close; John was a faster chugger than I was but I thought I'd keep him back if I could beat him out of the beer chug.

It was John, myself and another guy in the running for the win. The other guy finished chugging first, he took off, and then I finished and started chasing him. I caught up to him on the way out and beat him to the turn around. I was in first place and I could see the finish line! I was going to win! Then I felt a violent pile of gas in my gut make its way up. I thought I'd explode. I remembered the rule: "If you puke, you have to run an extra lap." I paused: false alarm, I pushed hard to the finish and then, "WHAM!!!" The other guy shot off like a cannon past me in a blur of tie-dye and huge compression socks. I tried to go faster but my stomach wouldn't have it. I came in second in 7:45 followed quickly by John.

Afterward, we watched as people puked themselves to the finish line. We went up to the house where they had lots of food, and we took a group photo and hung out with the rest of the Columbus Underground Racing Society.

CHAPTER 91

Leaving Columbus I could tell it would be a rather hot and humid day. I was right with both predictions. John knew of some short cuts cutting through a couple of neighborhoods and Fort Benning. This would cut off a couple of miles in the beginning of the run.

We spent most of the day talking about the year he did his Grand Slam of Ultra running and his run across Georgia which he would do in 3 days this year. We ran much of his route and he was able to tell me about some of the scenery as we passed and local stops such as the "Ranger Burger" at the restaurant that was named for the Army Rangers. We filled our bottles there and soaked our heads in the rising temperatures and humidity.

The hills rolled and we trucked along at the normal pace of 6 miles an hour. That was the day that I would be meeting up with my friend Dave who would join me for 5 days worth of running while pushing his own jogging stroller with his stuff in it. We were to stay at our friend Walker's inn in Marion, Georgia. As we came within the last mile or so, a police officer pulled in behind us turned on his sirens for a minute to pull us over. As he waved us over to the other side of the road, John and I looked at each other thinking, "What's this for?"

We stood on the side of the road and the officer got out of his car and walked up to us.

"So, what are you guys doing out here." We thought that was a pretty obvious answer but responded respectfully with, "running." He then prompted us for our identification in which John had forgotten being that he wouldn't be driving at all. This didn't go over well and the officer took my card back to his car to check me out. After several minutes he came back and in a semi-condescending voice inquired,

"I know you said you're running but what are you doing out here." I had to tell him about the cross country run and luckily John was there to vouch for me.

"Well, the reason I pulled you guys over is because I've gotten several complaints today about a couple of runners littering water bottles all over the road."

I was shocked. "Sir, I use this big Camelbak bladder, and two reusable hand-bottles. I don't carry plastic water bottles with me." He looked at John expecting an explanation, "Me too. I've just been carrying these two hand-held bottles."

He asked me, "Don't you have a case of water somewhere on this thing?" He pointed to my stroller like it was a contraption he hadn't seen before.

"Nope, just the Camelback and bottles. Are you sure they were calling about us? There were quite a few cyclists out today, maybe the caller was mistaken."

A tan SUV pulled up behind the cop car but we didn't think anything of it.

"No, every one of the calls said 'runners.' Well, here's what I'm going to do . . ."

Just then Dave pops his head out from the side of the car I couldn't see and says,

"Don't worry officer these guys aren't criminals." And he started laughing along with the officer. Dave and the officer shook hands all while laughing uncontrollably. Then a white haired man I could only assume was Walker came from behind the car laughing too. Walker's inn was across the street from the police department so he knew them all well. When Dave arrived at the inn he asked Walker if he could pull a prank on us with the local authorities. Walker was all for it and called his friends who were able to scare John and I enough to make it look real. They got us good and we all had a good laugh over it.

John, myself, and now Dave ran the last mile or so into town to Walker's inn, The Sign of the Dove Bed and Breakfast. It was a beautiful inn built in the early 1900s. Everything inside was wood and each room had a theme. After dropping off our stuff we all went to the local greasy spoon to chow down.

Soon it was time for John's wife to pick him up so we all took a couple of pictures and said our goodbyes.

The evening was spent catching up with Dave, getting to know Walker, getting Dave's jogger together and eating; always eating.

Chapter 92

The first morning with Dave, I woke up and packed our gear. When we went downstairs Walker had a huge breakfast for us all spread out—it was incredible! He said it was the "continental breakfast" but it was a beautiful spread full of anything you could think of. After Dave and I stuffed our faces, we finished packing our strollers, thanked Walker profusely and started off down the road.

Hearing Dave make the comments that I had thought when I first started made me realize how accustomed I had become to running on the side of a road with no shoulder. Things like, "Man! That truck was close!" or "This road slant is getting annoying," And the never ending, "Are we there yet?" I had forgotten how many times I had asked myself the same questions and made the same comments to myself at the beginning of this trek.

Our first day was pretty flat with the occasional rolling hill and had a sun that beat down on us like it was going to collide with the Earth. Dave's humor and characteristic chatting made the normal quiet road not so quiet. It was good to have company for more than a mile or two.

At around the halfway point we went through a town. Since we were unsure of the food choices in our ending town we decided to stop at a Subway and get lunch and dinner that we could bring with us just in case. We sat in the air conditioned Subway for a little while and recharged phones and ate our fill. While we were in there, a man came in who said he recognized me from TV and so we talked for a little while. Afterward, while we were still walking through the town, a van stopped and asked what we were doing. I told them and they said, "Yea! We saw you on TV!" And they gave me a donation right there on the spot.

Dave was impressed that people had just practically thrown money at me the whole way. I told him how much money people had really given me along the way in cash. I had hidden the money deep in my backpack but kept my personal money in my wallet so if I was robbed they would just take the wallet and not get the bulk of the cash for the fundraising. So far, I was up to about $750 in cash donations that I hadn't told anyone about. It was well hidden deep in my supplies. Needless to say, he was a bit surprised.

When we reached the town, we had heard there was a campground or RV park. Mixed messages from different people kept us guessing right up to the very end. The town was literally a strip of tiny shops that looked like a Wild West town. All of them were only open a couple of hours per day so by the time we reached them, they were all closed.

We did, however, find that the visitor center was still open so we went in and asked about a camp ground. It cost only $5 to tent camp overnight and they had a shower which, after the heat from the day, was very welcomed. She pointed us in the right direction which, unfortunately, was backwards, but only a bit. We found the grassy field and set up camp. It was nice to have a campground where I didn't have to arrive after dark and worry about being found.

We took turns showering and then had our leftover sandwiches for dinner while talking about races we wanted to someday run, long trails we wanted to run, and places we wanted to run to.

Lying in the tent that night staring at the yellow ceiling and walls that made up my tent, it hit me that I was almost done. I only had 11 days left and needed to start taking more days off because I was closer than 11 running days. I thought about how ready I was to see my family and my friends again. Even so, I had to admit that I had recently started looking at the north bound roads as more than just un-needed detours and instead as potential roads to take me to states I had not run through yet.

Physically, the running had become just something that used time. At the end of the day I was hungry but my legs felt fine. It wasn't difficult to complete the miles and I had settled into my pace religiously to the point where I could tell someone exactly where I would be at a certain time as long as I knew the mileage. Mentally, I was ready to see some of the familiar faces I missed.

CHAPTER 93

The second day with Dave brought with it 18 miles. It was very warm that day. We were fortunate to find a hose after 8 miles where we could soak ourselves and cool off for awhile. Straight roads and rolling hills made the day both interesting and pleasant. We ran by farm land and orchards but unfortunately there was nothing on the trees to pick. At the end of the day in Hawkinsville we made our way down the hottest and dustiest section of road I had seen so far. The sun baked us and zapped our energy.

Dave and I were picked up by a man named Kevin Collins. He brought us back to his house where we would stay for the next three nights. He was a large man, not in weight but in stature, and had a booming voice. He turned out to be really funny and when we met his family, they were very welcoming and fun. After getting cleaned up, I could tell Dave was tired because he fell asleep on the couch after sitting down for about 5 minutes. The Collins had three daughters who ranged in age from high school senior to preschool. Being an Italian family, they shared their family recipe of pasta with us that night and it was incredible.

The next day was spent sans stroller and was a relatively quick day of 18 miles, just as the day before. We found another hose to cool off in after several miles and it was a welcomed surprise.

Since we had decided to push the finishing date back at the beginning of the run so we could be sure that I would be there "on time," I now had a couple days off to burn up, the following day, was one of those days. We spent the morning on the Collins' boat on Lake Tobesofkee and it was the first time I had ever gone water skiing in early April. The water was calm and a little cool in the morning and throughout the day didn't actually change much.

That afternoon we went back to the house and relaxed for a little while until the girls got off from school and then we went back out on the boat where we spent our last evening with the Collins family. We went to the Fish'n Pig for a farewell dinner, a restaurant right on the water that had some killer hush puppies. The Collins family helped Dave and I enormously. Taking two strange men in was very trusting of them, and cannot fully express my gratitude for all of their help.

Chapter 94

From Eastman to Alamo, GA Dave and I had some interesting people interactions. We had completely forgotten that we had done a roadside news interview for channel 13 and apparently, a lot of people watch that news channel. We weren't 3 miles down the road and a van drove by going the same direction we were. It hadn't caught our attention until it turned around and started driving toward us and then pulled off onto the shoulder of the road. As we approached the van, a man got out and was holding a plastic bag. He waved and we stopped because he looked like he wanted to talk to us. The man simply said, "Hey, I saw you on the news last night, so here is some Powerade." We were a bit shocked but appreciated the gesture and thanked him. He was in a hurry so he had to leave before we were really able to talk to him.

From that point on that day, more people honked and waved then ever before. It was kind of cool but some of the people I couldn't tell if they were waving out of recognition or waving for us to get off the road because it was a heavily traveled road.

Another run-in we encountered was a motorcycle rider. He pulled the same maneuver the van had and again waited for us to get to him. Full on HOG rider. As we approached him, I have to admit I was anticipating some trouble. He was a rather large man riding a Harley with a leather vest and patches with "Born to Ride," "Loud pipes save lives," and "Ride or Die" all over it. He would've had no problem roughing us up a bit if he wanted to.

He turned out to be a great guy who had also seen us on the news. He told us about his shop, Fat Boy Camo. The business was screen printing t-shirts and tuxedo rental. He and said if we stopped by, he'd give us shirts. Five miles down the road we came up on his shirt printing shop and stopped to talk with him some more. He asked us about where we were staying that night and we told him we were camping in Alamo but didn't know where. Thankfully, he knew the people that own the funeral home in town, Townes Funeral Home. They let us not only camp in their yard, but also shower in the home.

I felt very refreshed and preserved after showering there. Maybe they mix the water with the preservative the Egyptians used . . . . But then again, maybe not.

That evening, Walker, the man whose inn we had stayed in the first night with Dave, was passing through the town we were in and picked us up and took us out for dinner. It was great to see him again.

CHAPTER 95

The next day marked five days left: a normal work or school week. It was hard to think about the fact that I only have that long until I had finished crossing a country on foot.

Waking up the last day I would run with Dave, I realized I didn't have to take things one day at a time anymore. I only had 102 miles left. I had run more in a 24 hour time span and it was a bit tempting to just finish the distance in one fell swoop.

The last running day with Dave was spent running to Vidalia, home of the Vidalia onions and they don't let you forget it.

It was great running with Dave that week. He's a tough guy who kept up with no problems, at least none that he told me about. I have to admit, I was a bit nervous about him picking up day after day of longer distances. He doesn't normally run everyday but he did great.

CHAPTER 96

I started the next morning in slightly cooler weather. It wasn't long until I passed a very familiar road, which was strange considering I had never run across the country before. It was Route 1.

I knew exactly where this road would take me. If I took this road straight north for a couple hundred miles it would take me three miles from my house in Stafford, Virginia. I had driven on Route 1 so many times and never gave it a second thought. In training for the run I ran from Richmond, VA to Stafford, VA all on Route 1. 70 miles overnight while pushing the baby jogger; I knew the road well.

In the 40s, my grandpa Pete McGlade drove the entire length of Route 1. Not all of it, if any, was paved and he passed the exact spot I ran today, just 60 some years apart. Let's just say it was hard not to turn north.

I ended in Claxton, which by the way is the fruitcake capital of the world. I was stoked! So I went into the store that said it baked the famous fruitcakes and bought one. The thing is, I don't like fruitcake, and I had forgotten that. That evening I stayed at a donated hotel room in Claxton.

Chapter 97

I was down to three days. A long weekend. Leaving Claxton was very difficult not to just keep running straight to the beach. But then again, because quite a few people were planning on coming down I didn't want to kill it for them since they were driving long distances to support me. Because of this and the fact that I had nothing set up for the evening as far as a place to stay goes, I was on my own for the evening. Since I wasn't meeting anyone, I took my time getting "where I was going," which I didn't actually know where it was. I stopped for a long lunch at Subway and continued on down the road.

Toward the end of my day I stopped into a convenience store and asked if there were any campgrounds or anything around. Of course there weren't but I continued on hoping to be so fortunate to find at least a solid piece of land to set up a tent on. Unfortunately, there were swamps all around and there was no way I was going to be able to camp underwater unless I sprung gills.

As it started to get dark I began to think that I was going to have to keep going until it got completely dark and then just start knocking on doors because of all the swamps. I passed a school and thought that as long as I was out by the time the first teacher got there in the morning it might not seem too creepy but it wasn't quite dark enough yet, so I kept going. Another mile or two down the road I ran by a fire house and the fire fighters were outside washing the trucks. Win.

I went up to them with my jogger and gave them my predicament. They said they didn't mind but they would ask the chief if I could camp out next to the firehouse. After a few minutes, one of the fire fighters came out and said I would be allowed to post up next to the fire house and if I was hungry they were making lasagna pretty soon. They also allowed me to shower in the fire house.

Of course, who was I to turn down any of their offers? I set up my tent, took a shower and joined them inside for some lasagna. I hung out with them for a little while before realizing I was semi-exhausted and went back to my tent for the night. They warned me that it was supposed to thunderstorm that night and just as I started fading off to sleep, a faint roll of thunder clapped in the distance and rain started to tap the outside of my tent. The pitter patter of the drops lulled me into a deep sleep and I was able to sleep all through the night, which hadn't happened in quite awhile.

CHAPTER 98

My alarm woke me the next morning but probably could have slept for another couple of hours. The rain was light and I didn't want to get up, but then again, I was running to Savannah that day and I was eager to get there. The firefighters that had been there last night had already switched shifts, so it made it slightly awkward to pack up my stuff because no one on this shift knew me. I tried to do it relatively quickly.

Moving down the wet street, my stroller's wheels made a quiet steady hissing sound that lent itself nicely to the early morning cool fog that gave the street an eerie feel. I ran strong and quickly out of anticipation of being in a city I recognized and being in a city that was so close to the end. After running along a road that had sand on the sides and a road that was back to being incredibly flat, much like most beach communities on the East Coast, I crossed under Interstate 95. Like Route 1, I-95 is also a very familiar road to me.

Along the back roads of Savannah, I came across a turtle in the road. Ordinarily, I would've just picked it up and moved it to the side of the road, but I knew that this one was a snapping turtle, so I grabbed the nearest poking stick. I decided to document the rescue for scientific research and pulled out the iPhone to start filming. After many snaps at the stick, getting him safely to the other side of the road, me still having all my digits, a good video, not to mention a good five solid minutes of shameless fun, I proceeded with my daily skip.

While running the streets of Savannah on my way to that evening's donated hotel, I passed under trees that were covered in Spanish moss. Normally, I would have thought it hung eerily from the branches, yet today, it seemed to sway in the breeze like banners or arms that were waving and welcoming me to this last city before Tybee Island. I reached the hotel right in downtown

Savannah. I could smell the ocean. It felt strange to get there because I reached water. It's not the open ocean, but there is a huge port where giant ocean cruising ships are docked; so I knew this channel went directly to the ocean.

My dad and Aunt Vickie were going to be flying into Savannah that night. I was supposed to leave a key for them at the front desk so that they could get in without waking me up. I decided it would be cooler to go to the airport and meet them there, especially because they weren't expecting it. I thought about running there, but decided maybe a taxi would be the best choice of transportation.

I waited for their respective planes to come in and each walked off the plane as if they were in a trance. It was late and after traveling everyone is more tired than normal, so it was understandable. I was very happy to see them. I hadn't seen either of them since I left California and they were surprised to see me. All of us were exhausted. We flopped in the beds in the hotel room and fell asleep within seconds.

CHAPTER 99

My last day off was spent with my dad and Aunt Vickie. We all spent much of the morning walking around Savannah and seeing some of the local sights. That morning, I spoke with the last school, St. Francis Cabrini. I had spoken to so many schools along the way; it became second nature for me. My dad and Vickie came with us and seemed to enjoy it almost as much as the kids.

Plans to get some of the final preparations done brought us to Tybee Island. It was there we met with Steve Palmer, the man who had contacted us so long ago to help us put on a big finishing day. I was finally able to put a face to a name and email address. He welcomed us to his island and we spent the next several hours touring the island and talking about how the last day would occur. He brought us to some of the local eateries and, of course, the seafood was incredible.

We dropped by the police station to talk to them about the intricacies of the police escort and Steve let us in on a little story. He had contacted them awhile ago to request a police escort saying that a guy named Patrick McGlade was on his way to Tybee Island after running across the country and Steve would like an escort for him when he got there. They put him on hold and transferred him to another officer. The second officer picked up and asked Steve what was going on. After telling the second officer about me the officer replied with, "Okay, now what is his name?"

Steve stated again, "Patrick . . . McGlade."

"Alrighty, now what is he wanted for?"

"What do you mean?"

"What kind of warrants are out for his arrest?"

They had thought I was running from the long arm of the law all the way across the country and somehow, Steve knew that I'd end up on Tybee. Steve set him straight about what was going on and everything turned out fine.

That evening Dad, Vickie and I met up with Steve and the rest of his family at Huckapoo's. It was a great pizza place that had a bar inside and corn hole and other games outside. After a full day of making sure everything was going to be ready tomorrow we drove to the DeSoto Hotel where my mom, my brother, Kevin, my sisters, Colleen and Bridget, and grandma had just arrived. I was so happy to see them all we didn't want to go back to Savannah, but everyone was so tired, we decided that would be the best answer.

CHAPTER 100

So like I was saying in the beginning, I woke up early on April 23, 2010. I was in Savannah, Georgia and had only 18 miles to go until I was completely finished. Hardly able to comprehend the whole trip, I stared at myself uncomfortably in the mirror, gave myself a little approving head nod and went to retrieve my phone.

Katie would be calling soon. She, her roommate, Sam, and our friend, Lara had driven all night so they could be here to see me finish. They would be tired so when they arrived, Kevin, my dad and I would evacuate the room so they could sleep while I was running and then could meet us at the Tybee Island beach.

Sure enough, as soon as I left the bathroom, my phone went off, they were in the parking lot. In a sleepy fog, my dad and Kevin both asked if they were here, I assured them they were and left the room to go greet them. They were understandably exhausted but it was great to see them all, but especially good to see Katie. Since I had to get to the beach at 2 pm, it was still too early to start running, so Kevin, my dad and I went downstairs to have breakfast. While sitting there eating, and half paying attention to the news, I heard the news start talking about a runner who was running for 24 hours to raise money for his kids' school. I found it ironic that I heard about a person running for 24 hours on the last day of the run that started as an idea from when I was running for the same time.

Kevin and I hung out for awhile while my dad took a drive out to Tybee to pick up my sister, Colleen. She and my friend, Adam, were going to meet me at the bridge leading onto the island so that they could run the last 3 miles with me.

Kevin said that he would start running with me for the last day and stop whenever he got tired. When my dad got back to the hotel he picked Kevin and me up so he could bring us to the hotel that marked my stopping point two days ago, and where I would start the last leg of the journey. We arrived on the spot at about 10:20. That would be just enough time to make it to the beach at a 6 mile per hour pace with a little leeway just in case disaster struck. My dad and Colleen were standing there, and at about 10:27 Kevin and I proceeded to remove our shirts and started running. I have to admit; I was a nice bronze color and wasn't worried much about sun burn that day. Kevin, on the other hand, was ghostly white from being fully clothed all winter while Virginia was buried under multiple feet of snow.

Virginia usually gets a couple of inches of snow here and there, and maybe a good storm or two that gets the local kids a couple days off from school. That year was different though because it snowed feet at a time.

Of course, I made fun of him for a minute because, as brothers, that's what we do. It never really occurred to either of us that maybe sunscreen would be a good idea. Kevin used to run high school cross country and did fairly well at it, but his real specialty is lacrosse. He plays defenseman because he likes to hit people with metal sticks. Personally I think it's because he's a wuss and doesn't want to get hit with metal sticks. Because of his switch in sports, his running shoes were a tad worn out and quite frankly looked like they had been fed through a lawn mower blade. The sole of the shoe, or lack-there-of, was actually peeled halfway off. The upper mesh had holes in it so you could see his foot through the shoe.

Even the laces were chewed up.

Though there's really no telling what adventure sealed the fate of his running shoes, I guess I just assumed he had gotten hungry along the way and taken a couple bites out of them. When questioned about the sad state of his footwear he said, "Eh, they'll be fine." And that was that.

Kevin is also one of those freakishly good athletes where you can ask him what he's been up to and he cites activities that any normal person would not attempt and just shrug it off like it's all in a day's work.

One day I got a call from him and he was all excited because he had just run 20 miles on a whim without training. I asked him how he felt afterwards and he just said, "Eh, fine." The day afterwards he was a bit sore but who wouldn't be. He also gets it in his head to do something and doesn't get it out of there until he's accomplished it, such as doing 1,000 push-ups in a day.

When he was younger, he also decided that he wanted to be on the Olympic bobsled team. So, he found the coach's name online and emailed him back and forth for awhile. It wasn't until he asked my parents if we could move to upstate New York and be home schooled that he was brought back to some reality and decided it might be best to finish 6th grade first.

Since the finish of the run, he has qualified for the Olympic skeleton team and now resides in Lake Placid, New York where he trains with the team.

Regardless, we started on down the road running through downtown Savannah, Georgia under the shade of trees that were thick with hanging Spanish moss. Soon we would not be so lucky to have the constant shade, and I doubt either one of us appreciated it while we had it. After about 3 miles we were in direct sunlight, and it was heating up nicely. The scenery of downtown disappeared and we were along a road that had sand on the sides of it.

Two miles later, we saw Dad and Colleen pulled over offering water. I refilled the hand bottle I was carrying; we doused ourselves nicely and proceeded down the shade-free road. I really enjoyed running with Kevin. Though my little brother outweighs me by about 20 pounds of pure muscle, we are about the same height and have a very similar stride. Apart from just going for a run like today, he also makes a great pacer for longer races because of our unspoken camaraderie. It was getting hotter now, and we were just catching up, joking around, cutting up and squirting each other with the water bottle as a way to stay cool and because we didn't have Super soakers available to us.

At 10 miles, Kevin had another chance to stop running and get in my dad's air conditioned car. He declined and said he felt fine to keep going. Parting from the car the last time, we started over the bridge that would take us to the flattest straightest section of road I had seen in quite some time. The road looked like it had been laid on top of sand and the sand was just floating in a salt water marsh. There was water all around us and there were only shrubs that grew wildly to keep our eyes occupied. The sun was very strong and beat on our shoulders and chests like we had insulted its mother. Again, Kevin kept trucking along never complaining about a thing except a bit of a stomach ache. I realized that we were going to get to our spot at the bridge where we would meet Colleen and Adam way earlier than expected if we kept up this pace, so we decided that we would rather walk and keep moving than to get there and have to wait. So that's what we did. Kevin's stomach was really bothering him so walking felt better to him anyway. He was a bit afraid that he "wouldn't make it" to the beach without finding a bathroom, so walking was definitely a good decision.

As we were crossing the bridge onto the island, we heard a car coming from behind us and they were honking wildly and yelling at us. I turned around just in time to see my friends barreling down the road arms flailing out of every window. Mike, Mitch, and New Tyler (we call him that because we had a friend named Tyler for years before the new Tyler moved to Virginia) had driven all night from Virginia and gotten to the beach only about an hour before I finished. While Kevin and I were walking down the other side of the bridge we saw the car my dad was driving pull up with Colleen, Adam and an unexpected Thomas inside.

Since we were still early, we went over to the side of the road to wait for the police to arrive. I set up my stroller because now I had plenty of room on the side of the road to push it now that we were going to have a police escort. When they arrived, there were far more than I expected. Four cars came out so I would have one in front and three behind so one would stay there all the time and the other two could trade off blocking intersections when they needed to.

The time finally came to run the last 3 miles and we all started out. Within 5 minutes, Kevin said, "I think I might explode." He ran off the side of the road to ask one of the officers where a bathroom was. We kept going because we weren't sure there was one. Surrounded by cops and listening to Adam sing random 80s pop songs, we ran down the unsheltered road toward the beach. About 10 minutes later we see Kevin sprinting up from behind us with a big old grin on his face. We couldn't help but laugh. He said, "I went to the cop and asked him where a bathroom was. He just said, 'The woods boy!' So, I went in the woods and then he drove me back up here." Since we were only taking up one lane of the two lane road, cars were still able to pass us on the left. As one drove by someone yelled out the window, "You cheated!!" at Kevin.

The sun still beat down on us all relentlessly and the salty air was making my skin feel sticky and heavy. Humidity combined with the rising temperature made it somewhat difficult to breathe but no one really complained. As we got into more populated parts of the island we started seeing marquis with "Run Patrick Run" on them and people were outside waving to us as our parade made its way at 6 miles per hour down the road. We finally made the sharp right turn to run on the street that paralleled the beach. My cousin, Chris, came out to join us but because he didn't know exactly what time I'd be there, had just inhaled a large burger and needed to stop soon after he started. It was good to have him while he was there though.

We made our way down the main strip and could smell the ocean. We were down to about 2 miles. Thomas said that his knee was bothering him a lot so he was going to, "Just ride in the cop car." Two minutes later, he ran back up to us.

"I opened the door and the guy just looked at me and said, 'Really? This guy just ran across the whole country and you can't finish 3 miles?' So here I am."

The officer behind us must have seen us laughing at Thomas and giving him a hard time because the police car let out a squeak and the loud speaker came on.

"Never say 'die!'"

We really laid it on thick after that.

As we ran passed a little Catholic school all the kids were outside and waved and cheered dressed in their uniforms and it reminded me of St. Francis, the school I went to, and did my practice run for talking to school kids. At about this time we picked up a few more runners. Some of them were kids, some were adults. I know for a fact that one was a teacher at the school because I asked her. I wasn't able to talk to all the people that were running with us for that section. When we ran by the YMCA (or middle school), there were some kids that were playing outside and two of them joined in our run just running in flip flops.

I took one more video for the blog and tucked my phone back in the backpack for the last time. One of the police cars raced ahead and took up both lanes and directed us to do the same. There were still quite a few runners with us when we made the final left turn to run down the two blocks of the street that led us to the wooden bridge that carried us over the sand dunes and inevitably to the ocean.

When we made the turn, I saw a lot of people on the sidewalks, but after about 5 seconds, they all turned into a blur. I don't know how fast I was running; I don't know who was right next to me at this point or who was directly behind me. I didn't really think about anything either. I pushed my jogger through the traffic circle and up the bridge.

Upon reaching the top of the bridge I could see the Atlantic Ocean. At the end was a giant arch that said, "Finish." The finish line was sponsored by Fleet Feet in Savannah so of course there were lots of those logos on it. Just beyond that were two paper finish lines held by some lovely bikini clad ladies that were recruited by Aunt Vickie spur-the-moment.

The bottom of the bridge led directly onto the sand and I left my stroller there in complete disregard, broke through both finish lines and ran toward the water. I remembered I had my shoes on so I tore those smelly puppies off along with my socks and just dropped them where I was. I made a straight line toward the water, saw my friends Mike, Mitch, New Tyler, and Mark on my left and didn't stop until I was fully submerged.

I was only underwater for a second but that second was enough time. Completely weightless under the water I saw nothing except the inside of my eyelids, but my brain populated my sight with a fast forward of my whole experience. Everything from the beginning, to the families I stayed with, to Grandpa's RV, the sights, the people, the secret family recipes, and the incredible kindness that was shown to me flashed by in that one second. A wave swept over my spot underwater and I was instantly brought back to reality. This is where I was, and this is the spot on the map where I pointed to so many months ago and said I would run to. Finding the sandy ocean floor beneath me I pushed my bare toes into the sand.

I stood up; made sure my shorts were still on, and I was then tackled by Mitch. Emerging from the water again I proceeded to hug my crying parents, my friends, and Katie. It was nothing like I had pictured it, and yet was everything I had hoped for. I had run across the whole country for kids with arthritis, and now was finished.

The problem was I didn't feel like I was done. It felt like I would wake up the following morning and run somewhere else, stay somewhere new and meet a new group of people. Sadly, this wasn't the case. My adventure had come to an end.

After half a million hugs and way too many pictures, the large group of people made our way back up the beach. Some went to get started on the plans for the evening party at Fannies. Some went swimming, and some went to take a nap, understandably. After a quick news interview I just kind of stood there; semi-lost and not fully aware. Katie came up next to me and I hugged her again. I had never been to Tybee Island before, but somehow, just knowing that I was on the East Coast and being surrounded by everyone I knew made it feel somewhat like home.

POSTSCRIPT

That evening everyone was invited to Fannie's for dinner. They had donated the third floor to us and we had a great view of the beach. It was very informal but was a nice close to the whole event. Several people spoke along with the mayor of Tybee Island, and I received my second and last key to a city. Everyone was so appreciative of everyone else and there were more "thank you's" than anyone knew what to do with. A little girl named Catherine spoke. She had arthritis and was one of the sweetest little girls I had ever met. Having her talk about arthritis brought pretty much everyone to tears and it reminded us all why we were all here. Finally it was my turn to talk. Before this event, I wasn't a very good public speaker. I wasn't very comfortable talking on a microphone and wasn't always so sure about what to say in a given situation.

I knew that I would have to talk at the end, so I thought about it long and hard, and I had quite a bit of time to think about what I would say. There were more people that helped me out than I could name. Even the ones I could name, I'm sure there would be people I left out so I decided to keep it simple and stick with the people that had been with me from start to end.

I thanked Steve Palmer for putting the whole finishing ceremony together and helping out so much with the local awareness of the event. He had no original ties to the event. He contacted us and offered his help as a local simply from the kindness of his heart. He didn't have to help us, or give us the time of day, but he did and we were all so grateful because of it.

All of my friends were due for a thank you. They had driven all night without knowing where they were really going or where they were going to stay. They had all called me at various times just to check up on me, and make sure that

I was still alive. Besides, they had thrown one killer going away party before the start.

Next on my list was my Aunt Vickie. She went way above and beyond the call of "auntly" duty. She promoted the run from the start in California and did so much for me without me asking her to. With an incredibly busy life as is, there was so many reasons she could have come up with not to help me, and quite honestly, I wouldn't have blamed her. But that wasn't the case. I couldn't image what the run would have been without Aunt Vickie the Great.

Katie helped me more than anyone knew and anyone could possibly understand. From the very beginning of the idea of this endeavor, she supported my ideas and never doubted me . . . that I knew of. On the tough days she told me I could do it, reminded me why I was doing it, and helped build up my confidence. On easy days, she was the familiarity that I missed about being home.

I thanked my mom. She kept me up to date with what was going on back at home and she kept my head level. All I ever talked about with anyone I met or came in contact with was the run. I liked talking to her because we talked about pretty much everything except the run. It was a good break and just felt normal to talk to her.

My dad was the last on my list. The run in and of itself probably wouldn't have happened without him. And the fundraising would have been minimal. He took on helping me as a second job and put in possibly more hours per week than his normal full time job. I am incredibly lucky to have a father who is as supportive as he is and the run would not have been the same experience had he not jumped in to help me.

After publicly thanking these people, a feeling of closure to this event came over me. It was over and I closed with the famed words of Forrest Gump, "I think I'll go home now."

They say, "Take some time to smell the roses," "Don't rush through things," and "Just relax and enjoy it." Although these old sayings might be clichés when it comes to everyday life, these are things that I lived by for 4 months while traveling. I saw a cross-section of America and met people who quickly became friends. They gave to me their help, money, resources and kindness. I believe this would not have been the same experience had I decided on biking or using some other form of transportation. I saw the country for what it is, and found a new side of people not many know exist; all because I crossed the country at six miles per hour.

Thank you to:

My parents, Desi and Susie McGlade, Grandpa Bob Muschek, Vickie Muschek, Katie, Mitch Young, Annie Tremper, Mark Davis, everyone mentioned in the book and those not mentioned who I stayed with, fed me, or donated to the run in any way.

Edwards Brothers Malloy
Thorofare, NJ USA
April 9, 2012